FUELLING THE FUNCTIONAL ATHLETE

Copyright © All Rights Reserved BOX NUTRITION 2020

Jack Braniff MSc. SENr. CISSN

All rights reserved. No part of this publication may be reproduced, stored in or introduced into a retrieval system, or transmitted, in any form or by any means now known or hereafter invented, electronic, mechanical, photocopying, recording or otherwise, without the prior permission of Jack Braniff.

Neither Box Nutrition nor any of its owners, trainers, affiliates, or associates of this system and all its publications, emails, forum postings, eBooks, website, and/or newsletters assumes any liability for the information contained therein. The information contained therein reflects only the opinion of the owners, trainers, affiliates, or associates and is in no way to be considered medical advice. Specific medical advice should be obtained from a licensed health care practitioner. Consult with your doctor before taking any nutritional supplement.

ABOUT THE AUTHOR

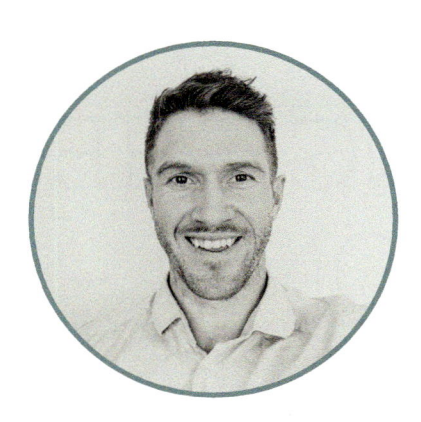

Jack Braniff MSc SENr

Jack has a Master's degree in sports and exercise nutrition, is a registered sports nutritionist (SENr) and a member of the British Dietetic Association (BDA). Specialising in endurance performance and functional fitness, he understands the difficulty in setting up a diet that improves both body composition and performance. Whether you are a competitive athlete or a recreational gym goer, this book provides you with the framework he uses to help his own clients achieve greater fitness success through better nutrition.

CONTENTS

What is Functional Fitness   9
1.1 What is functional fitness   10

Understanding your Numbers   14
2.1 Energy demands eating the right amounts   16
2.2 Macronutrients - The foods for fitness   31
2.3 Micronutrients   52

Fuelling your Training   57
3.1 Fuelling your training   58

Supplements   73
4.1 Supplements   74

Theory to Practice   82
5.1 Planning your diet   84

Scaling your Diet   96
6.1 The habit based approach   100

Calculate your Numbers   111
7.1 Calculate your numbers   112

Setting up MyFitnessPal   127
8.1 Tracking your food   128

Writing your Meal Plan   136
9.1 Writing your plan   138

Measure Progress   157
10.1 Self-assessment   158

Making Adjustments   164
11.1 Adjusting your plan   165

Your Prep Guide   173
12.1 Get prepped   174

Flexibility in the Diet   180
13.1 The balanced approach   182

Eating Out   189
14.1 Eating on the go   190

Meal Plans   196

Recipes   205

Resources   216

References   220

Glossary   231

"Nothing would be more tiresome than eating and drinking if God had not made them a pleasure as well as a necessity".

Voltaire

PREFACE

I decided to write this book after becoming frustrated with the amount of ambiguous, poor and often incorrect information that is spread by the host of unqualified influencers with regards to nutrition for functional fitness.

For me, it was plain to see how many recreational and even competitive athletes were failing to apply basic principles of sports nutrition to harness their performance and also improve the way they looked. The dogma attached to eating 'Paleo', 'Zone' and now 'Keto' as opposed to a personalised strategy has held back a number of athletes fulfilling their true potential. Instead, why aren't we taking well accepted sports nutrition practice from elite sports and applying it to this world of functional fitness?

This is the reason I decided to write this book. To break through the murky waters of nutrition for functional fitness, to use an evidence informed approach to breakdown and simplify exactly what is needed to perform and look your best.

How can we apply a number of fundamental scientific principles to improve all aspects of this discipline? Get stronger, fitter, faster, recover more readily and build a diet around making you a better functional athlete.

1

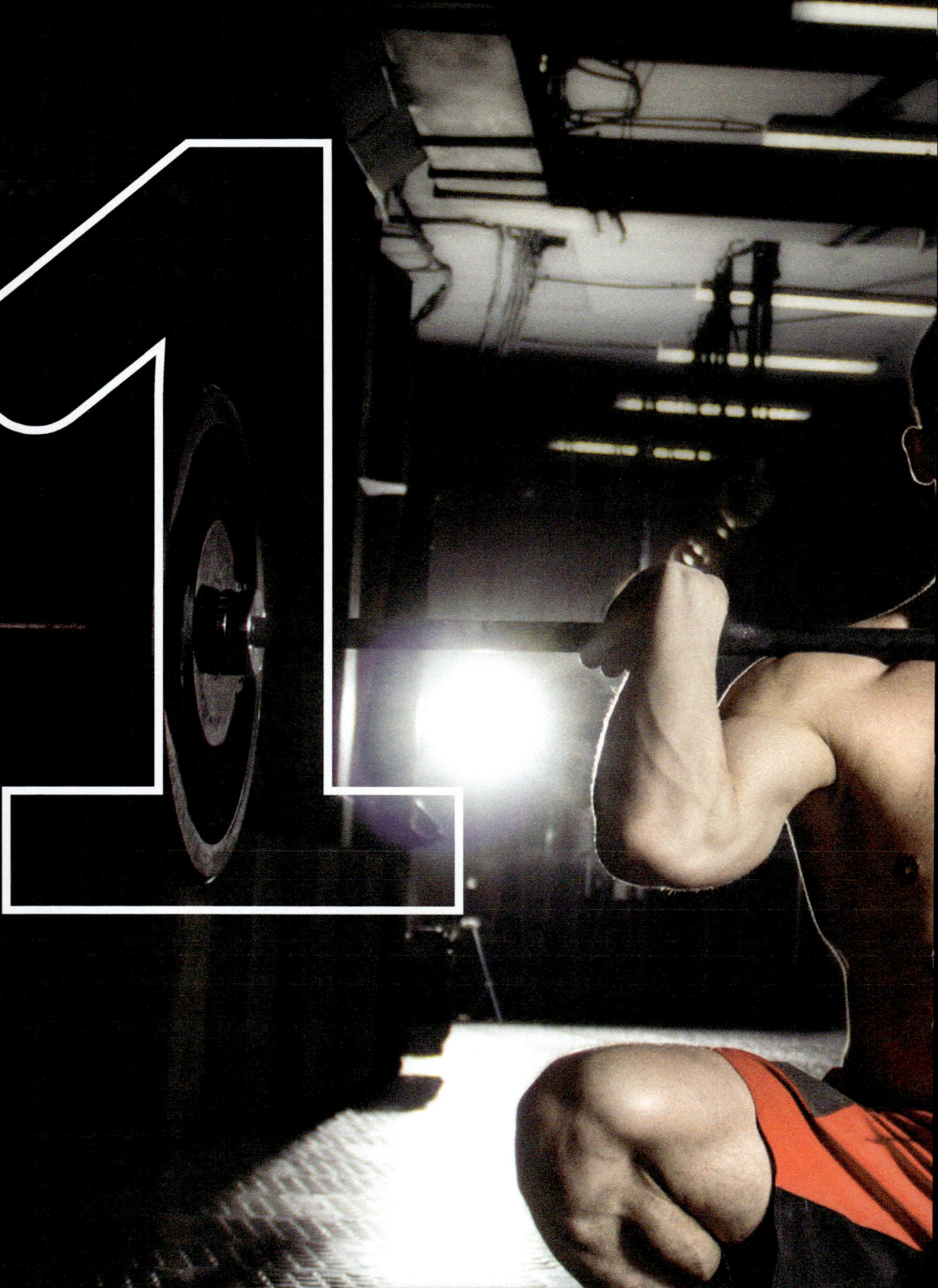

CHAPTER ONE

WHAT IS FUNCTIONAL FITNESS

1.1
WHAT IS FUNCTIONAL FITNESS

Although Functional Fitness is a very subjective and loose term, we can broadly break it down into the following areas:

- *Weightlifting (WL), which includes the major lifts (clean, squats, deadlift, presses and Olympic lifts)*
- *Aerobic capacity/metabolic conditioning/HIIT (cardio)*
- *Bodyweight exercises*
- *Gymnastic movements*

This list is not exclusive. Areas may be added or subtracted based on the angle from which you choose to view it.

Utilising this wide range of exercises, the idea is to help you improve capacity across the whole spectrum of fitness and exercise, as well as develop all three of the major energy systems (ATP- PCr, anaerobic glycolysis and aerobic system).

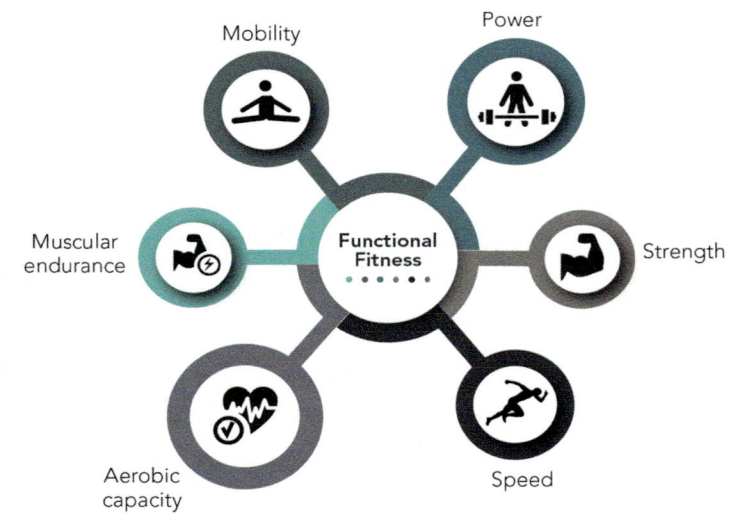

Metabolic pathways - Your Energy Systems

Metabolic pathways are the chemical and biological processes that provide energy to the body. By understanding these pathways and how each of them is fuelled, we can eat according to the demands of our metabolism.

1. ATP - PCr - This energy system provides bursts of energy for activities which require the highest amount of power, and typically last less than 10 seconds. Think of 100m sprints or Olympic weightlifting. This type of explosive activity can only be sustained for a short period of time on maximal output due to the limited ATP and Pcr stores [1].

2. Anaerobic Glycolysis - This energy system is used for activity which is prolonged for at least 1-2 minutes, but still produces a relatively large amount of power [2]. An example would be a 400m run or some of the shorter 'girl' CrossFit ® workouts that last around a minute with no rest, like Fran, Cindy and Barbara. This energy system works without oxygen, so lactate is produced. Although lactate is used later down the line as an energy source, it also results in an increase of hydrogen ions that reduce the PH of the cell. This inhibits force production and glycogen breakdown [2], which is why you can only maintain this level of force for a set amount of time.

3. Aerobic System - The aerobic system uses a combination of slow glycolysis, the Kreb's Cycle and The Electron Transport Chain. This third energy system will not provide the same power as the previous two, however it can produce considerably more energy over a longer period (several hours). The presence of oxygen allows more ATP (energy) to be produced and enable the exercise to continue [1].

Functional fitness looks to improve exercise capacity across all the components of fitness whilst, at the same time developing the three energy systems (ATP-PCr, anaerobic glycolysis and the aerobic system). However, depending on the workout, the contribution to overall energy supply will differ depending on intensity, recovery periods, duration of exercise and the fitness of the individual [3].

This is important to know, because, by defining the type of workout, you can manipulate your nutrition accordingly. Olympic weightlifting sessions will require adequate Pcr availability, highlighting the benefit of creatine supplementation. High intensity sessions that require the quick turnover of ATP will need more carbohydrates and beta alanine can help reduce the acidosis (hydrogen ion accumulation) resulting from ATP breakdown in the muscles. Low intensity workouts, in turn, can be fuelled by fat.

This further highlights the need to consider each training session in relation to the energy demand and intensity, so nutrition can be properly planned and structured. A flexible approach towards your nutrition will allow you to maximise performance, speed up recovery, prevent injury and improve how you look simultaneously.

This is the point where context and adapting your nutrition to the goal at hand becomes critical. A typical 'find your 1 rep max deadlift' workout will obviously require a different fuelling strategy to running a 10k. Therefore, it makes sense to view functional fitness as just an umbrella term, where more focus needs to

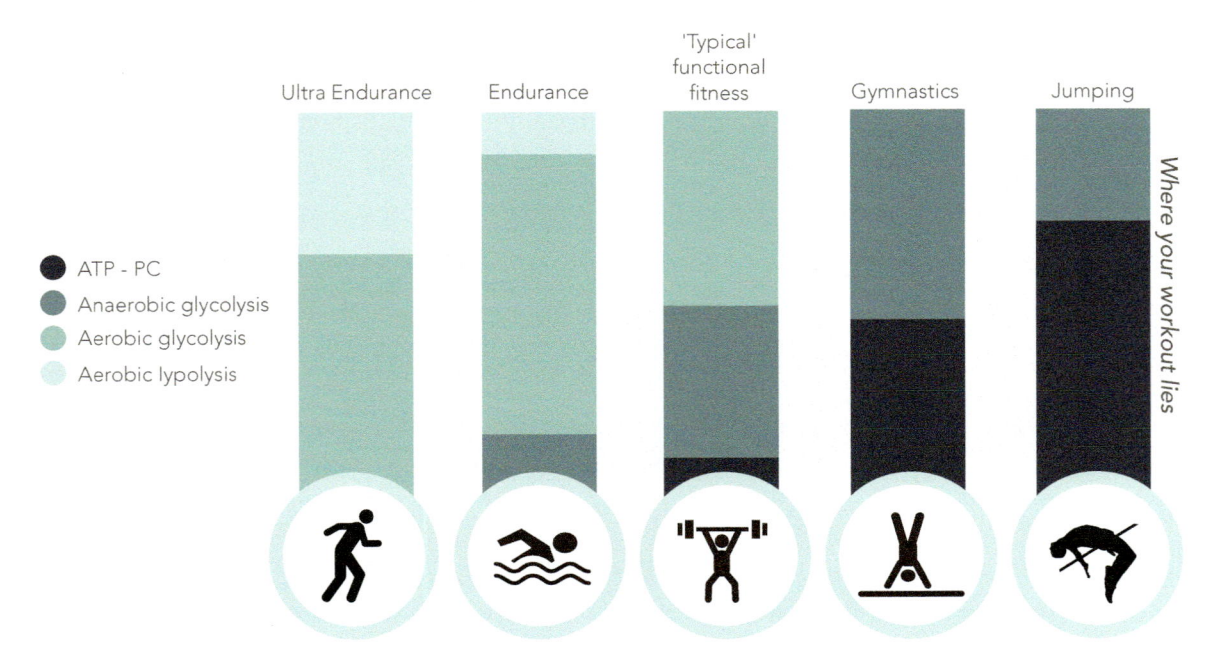

FUELLING THE FUNCTIONAL ATHLETE

be placed on its individual aspects, geared towards specific goals, rather than the sum of its parts.

Fuelling Brent Fikowski (2nd and 4th fittest man on the planet).

Brent Fikowski is regarded as one of the top CrossFit® athletes in the world, finishing 2nd and 4th respectively in the CrossFit® Games. For the run up leading up to the 2018 season, his dietician speaks of the importance of adjusting your food intake based on your energy needs and the work at hand.

"My biggest tip for sports nutrition is you need to change your food intake according to your activity level. Some workouts go for 10 minutes and others go for 45 minutes. You will need to refuel your body according to each workout! Don't fall into the trap of eating the same thing day in and day out!"

"So if Brent trains in the morning; he consumes more carbs then. If there is no activity at night he chooses lower carb options that are a little higher in fat. Protein intake never changes". Target Nutrition (2019)

This consensus of periodising your nutrition based on the activity is a common theme throughout this book, and is an important strategy to recognise to help develop your training.

As you would adjust your programme based on your needs, you must also adapt your nutrition accordingly.

CHAPTER TWO

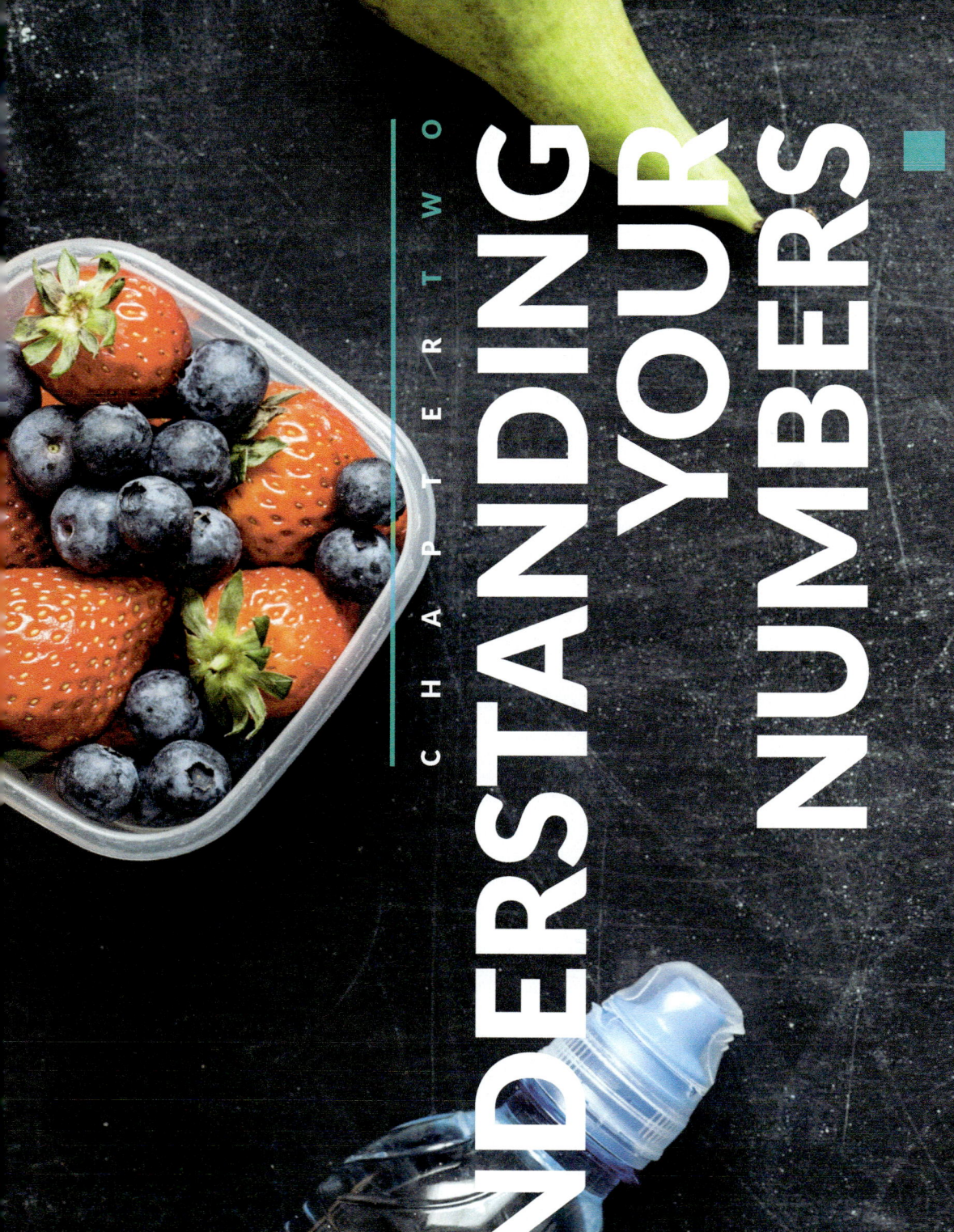

UNDERSTANDING YOUR NUMBERS

2

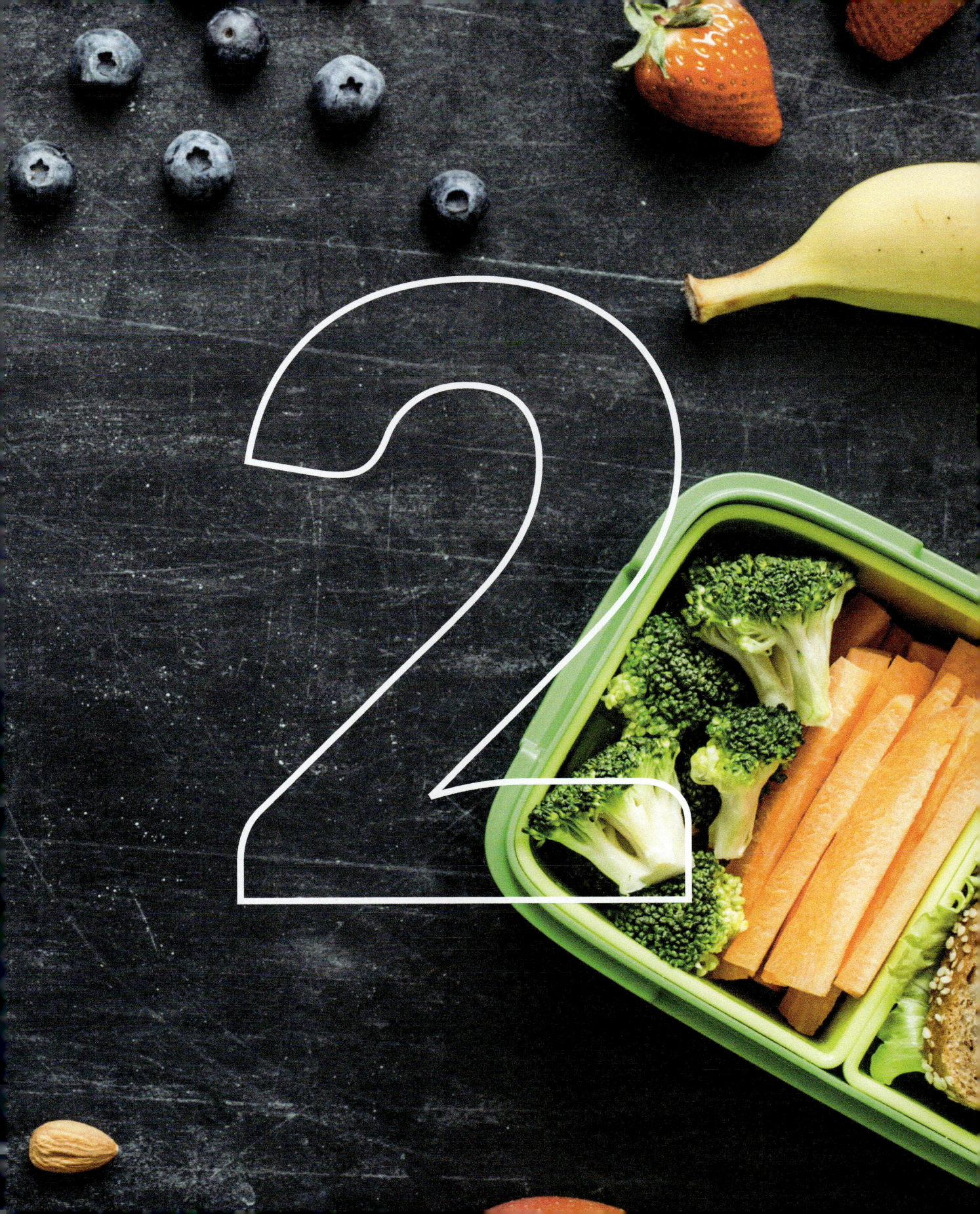

2.1 ENERGY DEMANDS
EATING THE RIGHT AMOUNTS

A proper diet that factors in the correct amount of food, correct food types, timings and essential nutrients should be fundamental for any functional athlete, whether your goal is performance, health or just to look good. A poorly designed diet that doesn't account for overall energy and the correct macronutrient ratio will blunt training adaptation, impede recovery, have an impact on energy levels, sleep, health and immunity. Eating the right amounts of the right foods is simply a critical step in becoming a better version of yourself.

Energy Balance

Energy balance refers to the food consumed through food and drink (energy in) compared the energy expended or 'burned' through activity (energy out). A negative energy balance or, kcal deficit, is when you expend more energy through activity than you consume through food. This will result in weight loss.

A positive energy balance or, kcal surplus is when you consume more food than you expend through activity. This will result in weight gain. Depending on your goal, you must look to carefully balance fuelling your activity correctly without causing fat gain.

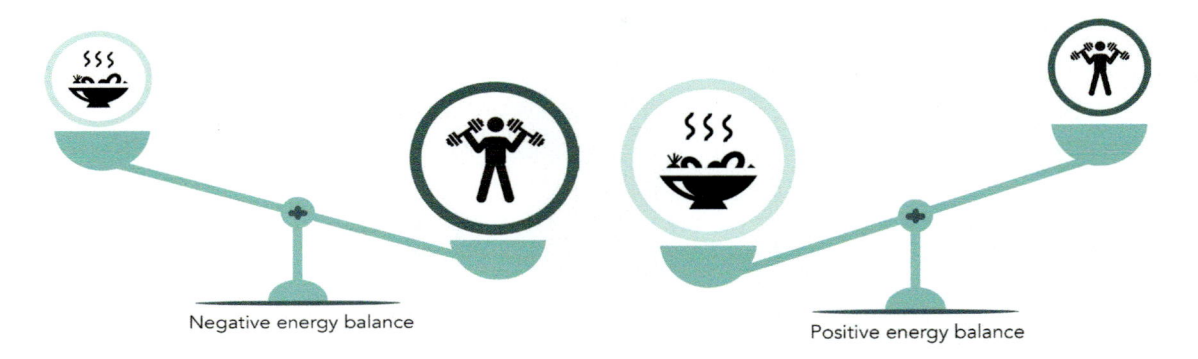

Negative energy balance

Positive energy balance

The effectiveness of your diet has will ultimately depend on the training plan you are following. For the average gym goer who trains 3 x per week for 30-40 minutes, following a 'good' diet will usually be enough to meet nutritional needs. However, for athletes involved in intense training of 2-3 hrs per day, 5-6 days per week may be expending 600-1200 kcals per session, then a well considered nutrition plan will be more important (1).

Individuals undertaking gruelling sports such as triathlon, long distance running, cycling, and any endurance athletes that are especially susceptible to a negative energy balance, will consequently increase the likelihood of unfavourable health and performance outcomes.

So where do we start?

Determining your energy needs

Energy requirements will depend on individual differences, goals, genetic make-up, age, height, weight, activity levels, training, and competition cycle. Your kcal intake should vary from day to day based on activity levels and intensity. How much you are supposed to eat can be determined by your total energy expenditure (TEE), which helps calculate how much energy you use in a day. This ensures you can eat enough to replenish the kcals your body will use.

This TEE is calculated by combining three elements of energy usage: the basal metabolic rate (BMR), the thermic effect of activity (TEA), and the thermic effect of food (TEF).

TEE = BMR + TEA + TEF

Test don't guess! - Metabolic Testing

As this method is still based on averages, the gold standard to calculate your RMR is through metabolic testing. If you were interested in having your metabolism or fitness tested, find out more and book your test at;

www.boxnutrition.co.uk/metabolic-testing

1. BMR

Basal metabolic rate refers to your body's daily energy expenditure at complete rest

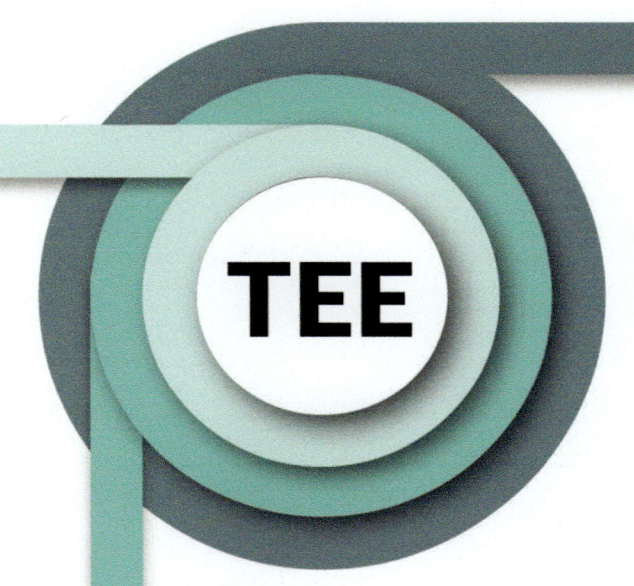

TEE

2. TEA

Thermic effect of activity simply means the energy cost of all physical activity. This includes non-exercise activity (like fidgeting) along with purposeful exercise.

3. TEF

Thermic effect of food refers to the extra energy your body expends to process and store the food you eat. TEF accounts for around 5-10% of TEE. As this number can vary depending on the type of food consumed and has such a small bearing on total energy expenditure, it is not worth being too concerned about.

Understanding Your Numbers

Calculate your BMR

You can use a simple equation to work out your BMR. Several methods exist, such as 'Mifflin-St Jeer', 'Harris-Benedict' or the 'Katch-McArdle' method. Although these methods may not be entirely accurate (calculations don't adjust for individual differences), it will at least give you a starting figure. We recommend using the Katch-McArdle method as it accounts for lean body mass. This is important because muscle is more metabolically active than fat, meaning it requires more kcals.

Katch McArdle Formula

BMR = 370 + (21.6 x Lean Body Mass(kg))

Mifflin St-Jeer Formula

Men: 10 x weight (kg) + 6.25 x height (cm) – 5 x age (y) + 5

Women: 10 x weight (kg) + 6.25 x height (cm) – 5 x age (y) – 161

Harris Benedict Formula

Men: 66.5 + (13.75 x weight in kg) + (5.003 x height in cm) – (6.775 x age in years)

Women: 655.1 + (9.563 x weight in kg) + (1.85 x height in cm) – (4.676 x age in years)

For a more accurate RMR reading, you can also use metabolic testing. Find out more at www.boxnutrition.co.uk/metabolic-testing.

FUELLING THE FUNCTIONAL ATHLETE

PAL

Calculating Thermic Effect of Activity (TEA)

There are two different approaches to help measure your TEA. The first and more simple method is to estimate the energy expenditure based on training volume, which is referred to as the Physical Activity Level (PAL), however, these figures can vary considerably due to a number of different factors, which is why they should only be used to give you a ball park estimate.

Physical Activity Multiplier

1. *Sedentary = BMR x 1.2 (little or no exercise, no training)*
2. *Lightly active = BMR x 1.3 (light exercise/sports 1-2 days/week)*
3. *Moderately active = BMR x 1.5 (moderate exercise/sports 2-3 days/week)*
4. *Very active = BMR x 1.7 (hard exercise every day)*
5. *Extra active = BMR x 1.9 - 2.4 (hard exercise 2 or more times per day, or training for a marathon, triathlon, etc)*

*Other PAL multipliers are available

HIIT

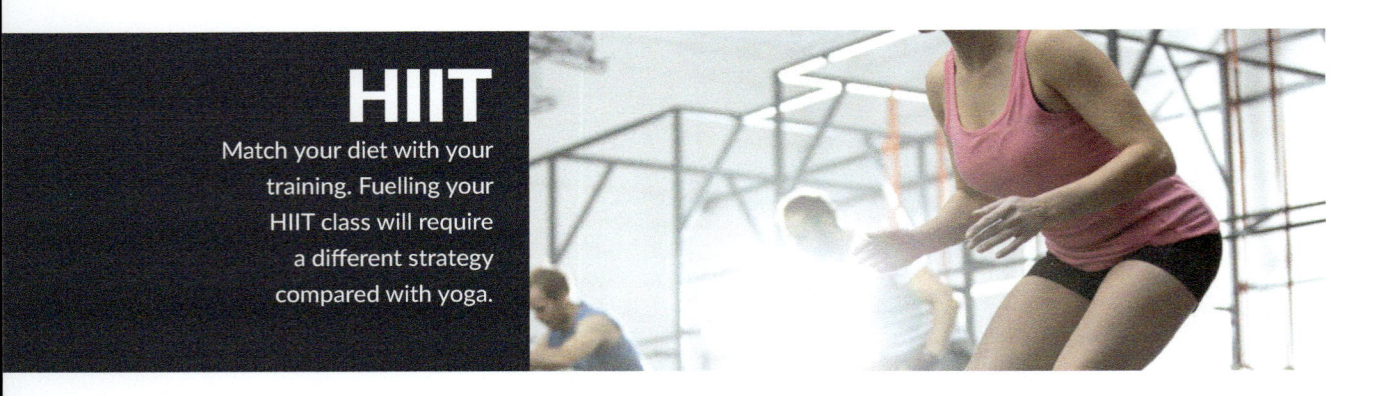

Match your diet with your training. Fuelling your HIIT class will require a different strategy compared with yoga.

Functional fitness can vary considerably from day-to-day where one session may comprise of Olympic lifting, to a day of only cycling.

The kcals expended during endurance training will differ greatly depending on you as an individual, the exercise, length and intensity of the session.

Strength and power training can be even more difficult to estimate because of the differences in volume, duration, recovery periods and type of exercise. Differences in muscle mass between athletes can also vary significantly, which will also impact the kcals expended during activity. Furthermore, considering the goal of most strength athletes will be to build muscle, they will need to be in a constant energy surplus.

For this reason, we at Box prefer to calculate your TEA based on your daily activity. By using activity codes and your weight, you can estimate your kcal expenditure from exercise to ensure you eat enough to perform at your best and properly recover. By multiplying your weight by the Metabolic Equivalent (MET) of an activity, you can estimate the number of kcals you will burn in an hour.

See Table 1. Kcal expenditure based on an 80kg athlete. For a full list of activity codes see the 2011 compendium of physical activities.

Weight - 80kg		
Activity	MET	Kcals per hour (weight x MET)
Running, 7mph (8.5 min/mile)	11.0	880
Running, 8mph (7.5 min/mile)	11.8	944
Swimming (vigorous laps)	9.8	784
Swimming (moderate effort)	5.8	464
Calisthenics (e.g. push ups, pull ups), vigorous effort	8.8	94.4
Resistance training, slow or explosive effort	5.0	400
Resistance training, multiple exercises, 8-15 repetitions	3.5	280
Circuit training, vigorous intensity	8.0	640
HIT training WOD Cindy	9.5	760
Rowing (moderate effort)	4.8	384
Rowing (vigorous effort)	6.0	480
Yoga/mobility	2.5	200

Table 1 - Taken from compendium of physical activities (Ainsworth 2011)

You could also cross reference this figure with a fitness wearable (like a smart watch or Fitbit®) to give you an idea of your energy expenditure for the day. Keep in mind that these fitness devices are often not entirely accurate (3), so use them only as a guiding estimation.

For the reasons listed above, your calculated energy expenditure will not be totally accurate, and it should only be used as a starting measure. The difficulty in calculating precise energy needs illustrates why the process of determining how much to eat must be fluid and adjustable. Metrics such as body composition, recovery, and performance in the gym should be used to modify dietary needs moving forward, rather than rigidly sticking to set nutrition guidelines calculated at the start (See Chapter 11 for more on making adjustments).

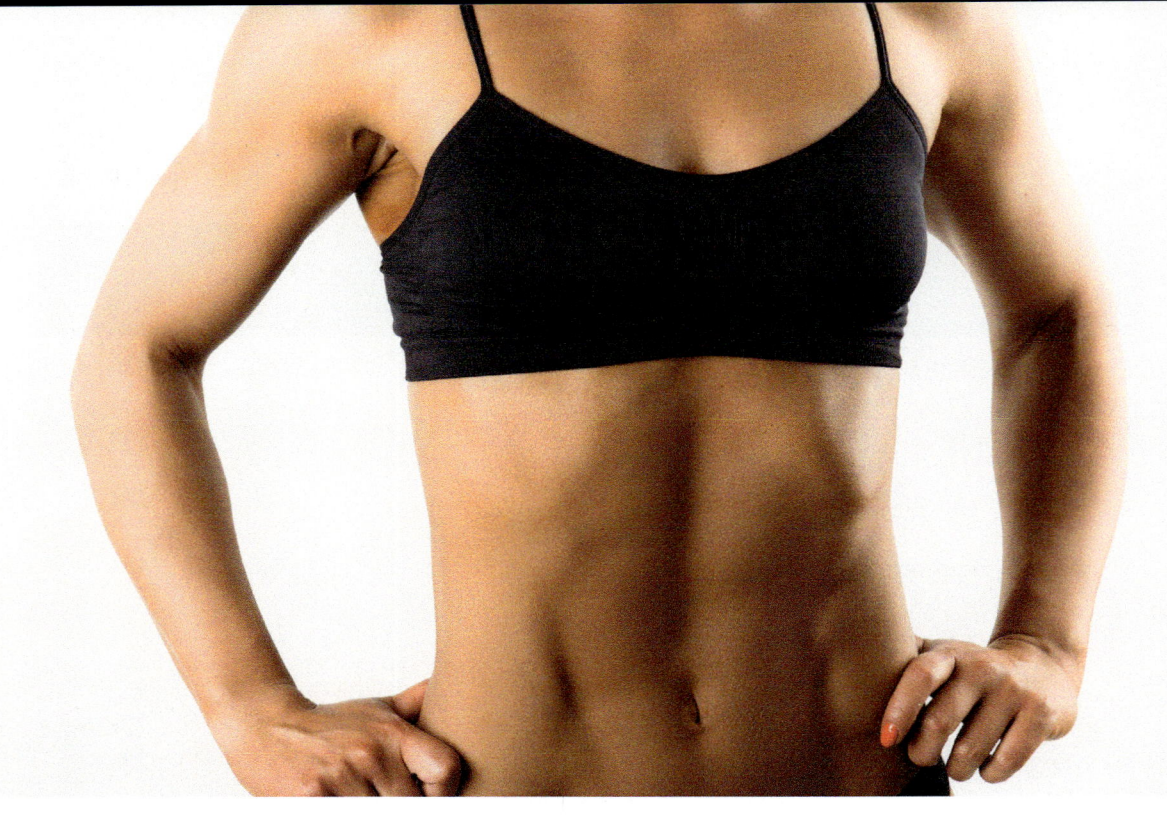

What about body composition?

Body composition is used to portray the ratio of muscle, fat, bone and water in the body. Better body composition indicates a higher percentage of muscle mass compared to fat mass. Better body composition is not just about looking good. Improved body composition will also:

- *Optimise power-to-weight ratio*
- *Make your body more efficient by reducing the energy cost of movement*
- *Increase speed and agility*
- *Allow your body to move within smaller spaces in some of your gymnastic movements (4)*

For athletes with heavy energy demands in both volume (a lot of sessions) and intensity, it is important to be prudent when trying to lose weight. An increase in training, a decrease in food intake, or a combination of the two can negatively affect performance and health. If your body composition needs improvement, a carefully periodised strategy over time is better than implementing a more aggressive short-term plan. Try and align your nutrition with your training and accept that there will be some fluctuations throughout the year.

RED - S

Energy Availability (EA) is a term that refers to the number of kcals you have left over, once you have accounted for the energy (food) you consume and the energy you have expended through activity. Low energy availability or Relative Energy Deficiency in Sport (RED-S), is a 'mismatch', or, being left with insufficient kcals for the body to be healthy and function correctly.

To calculate Energy Availability:

Energy Availability (EA) =

Energy Intake (EI) (kcal) –Exercise Energy Expenditure (kcal)/ Lean Body Mass (LBM) (kg)

A consistent daily energy availability of below <30 Kcal's.kg.lbm may lead to a number of adverse effects on health and performance, which include bone health, menstrual function, cardiovascular health and metabolism (IOC Consensus, 2018). A difficult concept to actually measure, athletes should instead be aware of symptoms associated with the condition and make a concerted effort to fuel their activities correctly.

Adjusting your kcals for weight loss

A sensible approach when trying to reduce weight is to minimise the rate of weight loss by creating a modest kcal deficit. This daily reduction should be around 250-500 kcals where bigger athletes should opt for a larger drop in kcals. You can also decrease your TEE by 15% (multiply your TEE by 0.85), or incrementally increase the number of kcals you expend through exercise (6). If performance is not important, then a more aggressive decrease of 25% can be implemented.

Adjusting your kcals for weight gain

If weight gain is the goal, then use a similar incremental approach to prevent unnecessary fat gain. A general rule of thumb is to increase your daily kcal intake by around 500-1000 kcals or by multiplying your TEE by 1.2 depending on how aggressive you want to be.

Like most nutrition strategies, the important point is to operate on a case by case basis where individual differences, goals, day to day training, competition cycle (eating for competition will be very different compared to your off season), preferences, and history should be considered. Continued monitoring and reassessment should be used to build a better long-term strategy.

Stay flexible and use recovery, performance, and body composition metrics to dictate alterations in your plan going forward (see Chapter 10 for more on measuring your progress). Try to err on the side of eating too much rather than not enough, since a decrease in performance is less desirable than a slower rate of fat loss. Increases in lean mass and improvements in strength, capacity, and speed will also contribute to favourable changes in body composition.

To sum up

1. BMR
Calculate your BMR using either 'Katch Mcardle', 'Mifflin-St Jeer' or the 'Harris-Benedict' method

2. Energy Expenditure
Multiply by your daily physical activity level (PAL) or use MET's and cross reference with fitness devices that record your energy expenditure through exercise to increase precision.

4. Adapt moving forward
Use recovery, performance, and body composition metrics to monitor and adjust your needs going forward.

3. Adjust for your goal
Adjust calorie intake depending on your body composition goals. If your goal is weight loss, reduce by 250-500 calories or multiply your TEE by 0.85. If your goal is muscle gain, then increase by 500-1000 calories per day or multiply your TEE by 1.2.

Understanding Your Numbers

The Reality of RED S

Anna Boniface was one of the top female prospects of British distance running after finishing the London marathon as the first amateur athlete. Her performance earned her a place on the England team, however, her international debut was cut short when her body broke down, literally. A stress fracture to her fibula ended her race and further tests highlighted an even worse picture. Anna had developed osteoporosis of her spine and her bone density was poor, symptoms of Relative Energy Deficiency in Sport (Red-S). Her actions over several years had taken its toll.

"Eating Disorders and the many issues around Relative Energy Deficiency in Sport are alarmingly common in running. We all know it exists, yet it remains a topic of taboo. Too many athletes are compromising their health for the sport they love without action being taken". "It inspired me and others to speak out about the dangers of undereating, over-training and the importance of periods". (Anna Boniface).

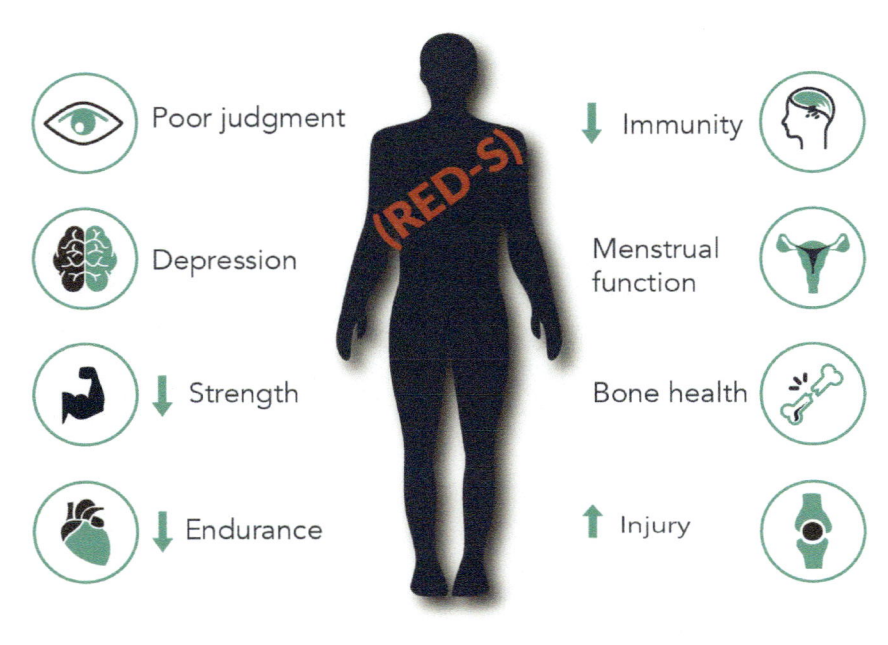

Symptoms of RED S

RED S is a serious concept and should not be taken lightly. Don't let it hamper your health and performance by under-fuelling your training. Recognise that exercise is not a punishment, losing your period isn't a normal consequence of endurance training and you shouldn't have to feel you need to earn food (Trainbrave.org).

#TRAINBRAVE is a campaign in the UK that aims to raise awareness about eating disorders in sports and help deal with issues related to RED-S. Train Brave's purpose is to provide resources and direct athletes to the appropriate services to deal with the issues related to RED-S. To find out more visit **https://trainbrave.org**

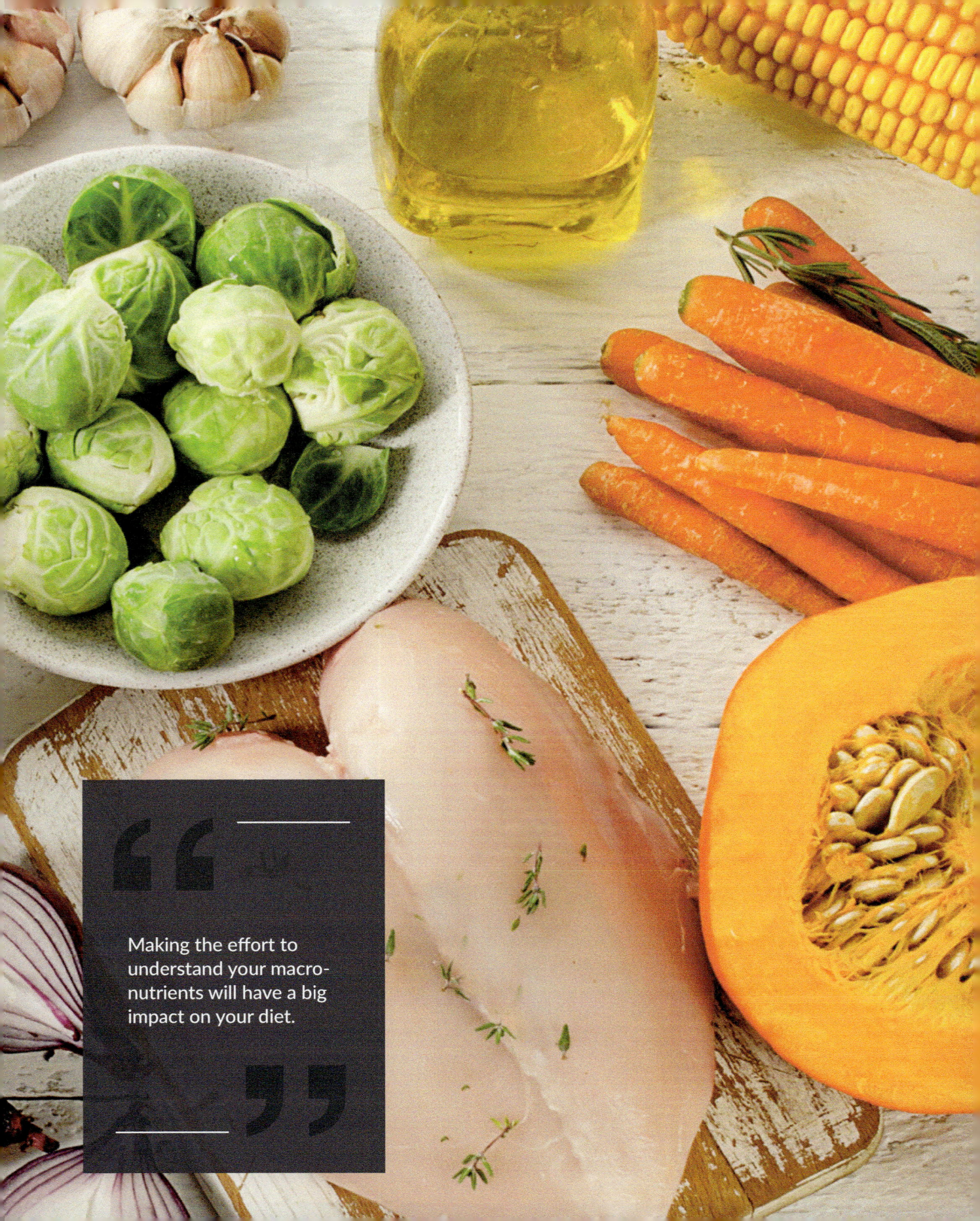

> Making the effort to understand your macro-nutrients will have a big impact on your diet.

2.2
MACRONUTRIENTS
THE FOODS FOR FITNESS

In addition to getting overall caloric intake right, functional athletes must also strive to consume the major food groups in the correct quantities. The right balance between carbohydrate, protein and fat is essential for optimal performance, recovery and body composition.

These major food groups are referred to as macronutrients or macros. They are the nutrients our bodies require in larger amounts and the ones that we draw energy from. Although not quite as important as overall kcals, a correct balance of macronutrients still considerably contributes to reaching your goal. Learning about types of macros, sources of different macros, and how to add them into your meal plan will have a big impact on fuelling your workouts and helping you achieve your performance and body compositional goals.

Carbohydrates

What are carbohydrates needed for?

Carbohydrates (CHO) are the main source of energy for the body and as such are responsible for fuelling both exercise and the nervous system (brain). However, overconsumption will lead to the development of fat deposits in the body. As athletes we must learn to balance our nutrition in a way that allows high. performance, but doesn't compromise body composition.

It is generally accepted that carbohydrates are vital for moderate/intense endurance exercise (>75% VO2max), HIT training and team sports, among others. (8, 9, 10).

Low carbohydrate diets such as Keto, Paleo and Zone diets are often associated with certain areas of functional fitness like CrossFit® (11). However, studies suggest that when exercise is performed at a high intensity, performance is inhibited when carbohydrates availability is low (12).

In this part we will dive into the science. I know it can be boring and slightly overwhelming, but it is crucial to gain an understanding of what happens in your body, so you can optimise both training and body composition.

During periods of low intensity exercise, the aerobic system (see p. 9) generates energy by using both fats and carbohydrates. During high intensity exercise, the aerobic system is unable to keep pace with the increased energy demands and the body has to resort to anaerobic glycolysis which uses only carbohydrates to generate energy.

Although workouts will utilise both aerobic and anaerobic pathways, the focus of functional fitness is to exercise at a high intensity, that is mostly using the anerobic pathway. It follows that performing well in these types of workouts will require enough carbohydrates (13, 14, 15).

What about longer moderate intensity sessions?

Recent guidelines (16, 17, 10) help make a conclusive argument that carbohydrates during lengthy (>2 h) moderate-to-high intensity exercise can significantly improve endurance and performance (18).

The case for low carb

In recent years, Low Carbohydrate High Fat (LCHF) diets have gained popularity; but why is this?

Fat, as a macronutrient, has a fairly large supply from body fat in the average human, greatly outweighing stored carbohydrates, in the form of glycogen. Glycogen is the carbohydrates stored in the muscles and liver. We can store roughly 100g of glycogen in the liver and around 400 g in the muscle (this will depend on the amount of muscle mass of the individual) (19).

LCHF diets can also increase fat oxidation (using fat as fuel) during low intensity exercise (<75% VO2max) (20, 21, 22). However, this is still less economical (less energy in the form of ATP is produced per ml of oxygen used) than carbohydrate metabolism and as such, is less able to support exercise requiring more energy and oxygen (>75% VO2max) (12).

Studies show that none of the theory about LCHF diets translates into improvements in performance for medium and high intensity exercise (23, 24). When highly trained athletes compete in endurance events lasting up to 3 hours, carbohydrate, not fat, serves as the main source of energy and fuel for the muscles. Studies have established that the presence of carbohydrates, not fats, become the limiting factor for performance (25).

As we will discuss later in this chapter, there may be some advantages of low carbohydrate training, however they will still be the preferred fuel for competition.

The area where LCHF diets may become advantageous is ultra-endurance. However, this is an area that needs to be considered in greater detail that goes beyond the scope of this book.

What about strength training?

Similarly to understanding how endurance training works, let us now take a look at strength training, so we can better understand the metabolic demands and how to fuel them. Resistance (strength) training varies considerably depending on volume, intensity, rest between sets, repetition tempo and other factors. Strength training can be broadly categorised into:

- *Low rep (less than 6 reps) at high intensity (at weight greater than 85% 1 Repetition Max (RM)) with longer rest periods (>3 min)*
- *Hypertrophy (muscle building) using more repetitions (> 8), moderate intensities (weights if 60-80% 1 RM), and shorter rest periods (< 2 min)*

Research suggests that glycolysis (the use of carbohydrates as fuel) is greater during hypertrophy type sessions using higher volume (volume refers to the number of muscles worked, exercises, sets, and reps during a single session). This means that glycogen, the carbohydrate stored in the liver, blood and muscles, will reduce. This reduction in muscle glycogen can lead to reduced force production, which in turn affects performance in a strength training session (26). Glycogen stores will not fall as much with lower volume strength and power training (27).

This means that more carbohydrates are required for a greater volume of work (number of reps and sets) at higher intensity (reaching until failure) when muscle building is the goal. Maximal strength and power sessions do not require the same amounts (27). However, increasing blood glucose (sugar) prior to shorter types of sessions can still help with increasing volume, duration and strength. So, a small amount of carbohydrates before these types of sessions will be beneficial.

What fuels your activity

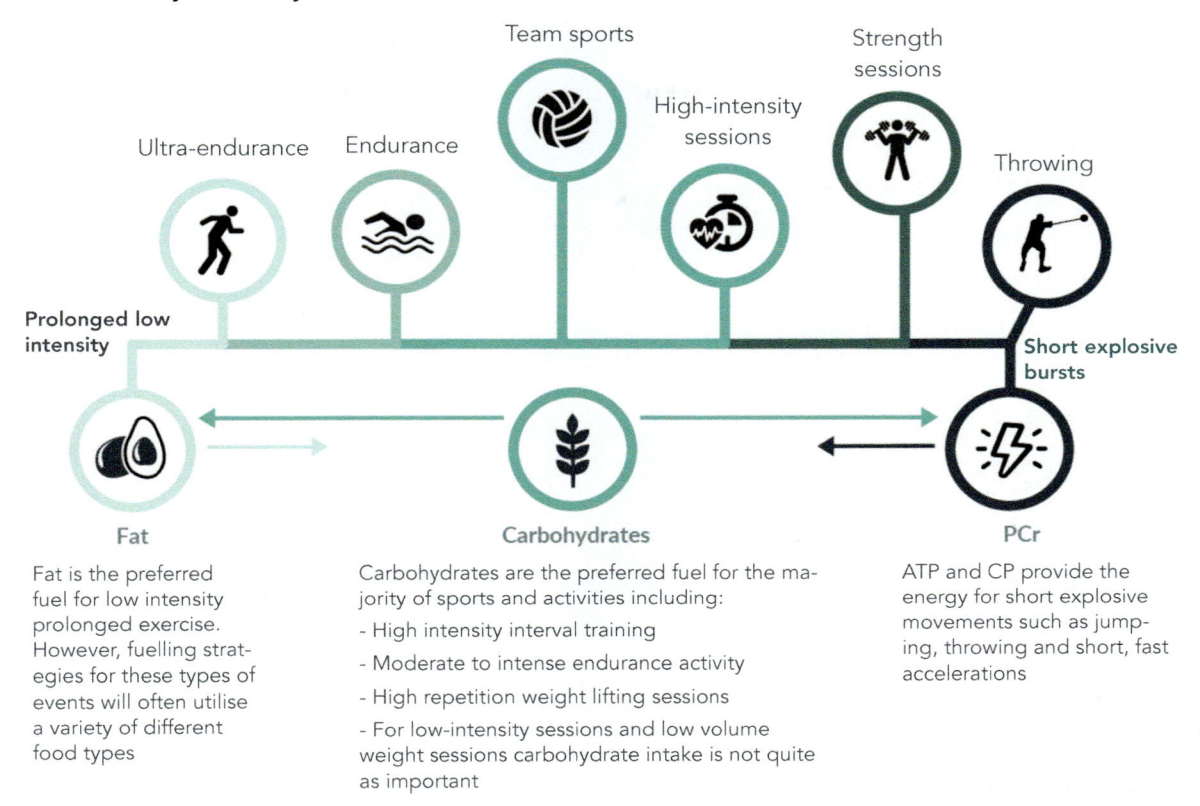

```
Prolonged low                                                              Short explosive
intensity                                                                  bursts
  Ultra-endurance   Endurance   Team sports   High-intensity   Strength    Throwing
                                              sessions        sessions
       Fat                      Carbohydrates                              PCr
```

Fat is the preferred fuel for low intensity prolonged exercise. However, fuelling strategies for these types of events will often utilise a variety of different food types

Carbohydrates are the preferred fuel for the majority of sports and activities including:
- High intensity interval training
- Moderate to intense endurance activity
- High repetition weight lifting sessions
- For low-intensity sessions and low volume weight sessions carbohydrate intake is not quite as important

ATP and CP provide the energy for short explosive movements such as jumping, throwing and short, fast accelerations

What does this actually mean?

- Because of the great diversity in functional fitness, your carbohydrate needs will be dictated by the type of exercise and training
- Adequate carbohydrates are needed to perform well when training at a high intensity, moderate to high volume for sessions shorter than 2 hours. For low intensity and low volume sessions, they are not quite as important
- Finally, how many carbs you need will depend on you, your training, goal and preference

Understanding Your Numbers

What does g.kg.bw mean?

We use this terminology to express how much of a particular food, liquid or supplement we require. For example. If we require 2 grams of protein per kilogram of bodyweight, we would say 2g.kg.bw. If we require 5 millilitres per kilogram of bodyweight we would say 5ml.kg.bw.

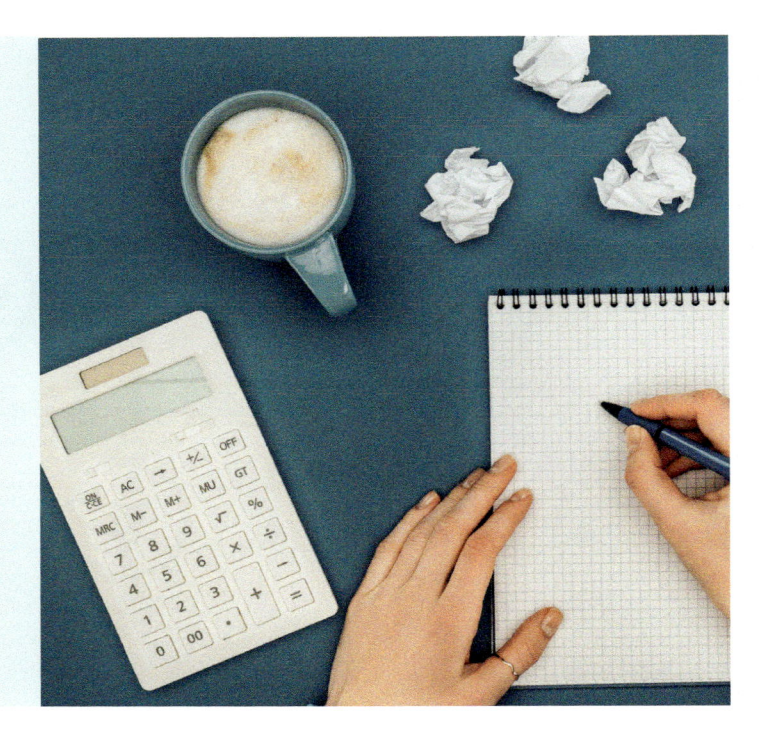

So how many?

One of the most important factors to proper nutrition is finding the right balance between eating to fuel your workout without leading to fat gain. Even though textbooks may recommend a carbohydrate intake of 6-10g per kg of bodyweight per day (which is a lot!), smaller workouts and rest days will obviously require less. On the other hand, training twice a day or working the same muscle group on consecutive days will require a far greater quantity.

Research has not shown a clear advantage of high carb diets over moderate carb diets concerning performance (28). That being said, no negative consequences have yet been associated with a high carb diet. So, if performance is the goal, athletes should normally aim or, at least steer towards, a higher carbohydrate diet (3-7g.kg of bodyweight per day). This will ensure performance is maintained at a high level. While it is true that resistance training utilises glycogen as its main fuel source (25), total caloric expenditure of strength athletes is less than that of mixed sport and endurance athletes. Thus, authors of a recent review recommend that carbohydrate intakes for strength sports, including bodybuilding, should be between 4–7 g.kg depending on the phase of training (16).

Carbohydrate periodisation

The concept of *fuelling the work required* helps us decipher how to adjust carbohydrates based on training and activity. How many carbohydrates you actually need will be dictated by the type of day and type of exercise you are doing. Amounts of carbohydrates should be defined by the goal of the athlete, their body weight (size of muscle stores), the type of the training sessions, training volume, and intensity. The more training you do and the more muscle you have, the more carbohydrates you need.

Similar to how you would periodise your training programme, carbohydrate intake can also be periodised. This can be based on different training blocks, different days and can even change over a 24hr period. As with kcals, you should not adhere to a set number; rather *"change between categories according to daily/weekly/seasonal goals and exercise commitments"* (16).

Daily Carbohydrate Needs

Athletes involved in low volume powerlifting or Olympic weightlifting will not require more than 1.5-3g.kg.bw per day to support training and recovery. For athletes who train 1-2 hrs per day and take part in a general fitness or gym programme, the typical carbohydrate recommendations (i.e. 45–55% or 3–5g.kg.day) will be enough to fuel endurance sessions under 60mins, high intensity interval training and high volume resistance training. However, those involved in high amounts of training (2-3 hrs per day) will need to consume up to 5–8g.kg.day of carbs. For athletes participating in very high amounts of training (3-6 hrs per day) the carbohydrate needs may be up to 8-10g.kg.day (1, 38, 16).

Rest days will come down to the athletes' preference and overall energy requirements for the day. This should fall somewhere between 1-3g.kg.bw.

CARB Recommendations

Very Low — Rest day
1-3 g.kg.bw.d

Low — Low volume strength training - Powerlifting/Olympic weightlifting. Gymnastics
1.5-3 g.kg.bw.d

Moderate — Metabolic conditioning. HIT training. High volume resistance or circuit training
3-5 g.kg.bw.d

High — Aerobic capacity /endurance work/training twice per day. 2-3 hrs per day.
5-8 g.kg.bw.d

Very High — Very high. Extreme programming. 3-6 hrs per day
8-10 g.kg.bw.d (3-6hrs)

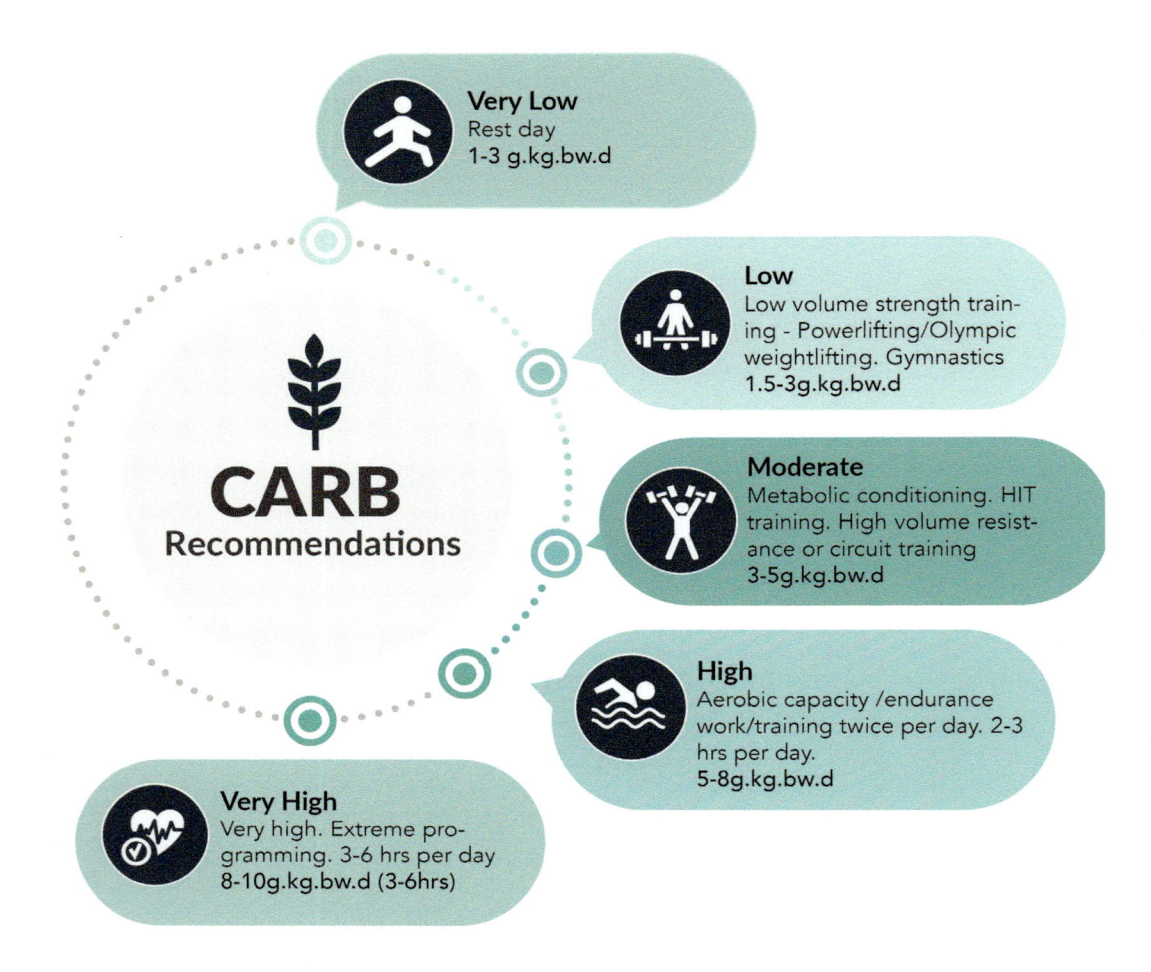

Carb recommendations

These numbers are only a starting estimate and need to be fine-tuned and personalised using a 'trial and error' approach based on performance and body composition metrics.

Training Low

A concept growing in popularity is "training low", which refers to commencing exercise sessions under low carbohydrate availability. Restricting carbohydrates helps activate the protein PGC-1 alpha that can increase the number of mitochondria (the power plant of the muscle), the density of small blood vessels (capillaries) and density of slow twitch muscle fibres. These effects can provide a benefit to endurance performance (29, 30, 31). Although carbohydrates alone don't have a direct impact on weight loss (total caloric intake and expenditure, or energy balance, does), recent research suggests that this type of training improves fat oxidation over a period of time, independent of total energy balance (32, 33). From this it is possible that when weight loss is your priority, training "low" could be a useful strategy to help become more efficient at using fat during exercise. This is because an increase in mitochondria enables more oxygen to be used for energy, increasing the intensity at which you are able to use fat as a fuel source. However, these adaptations can also be brought about by improving fitness, highlighting how 'train low' is just a small piece of the puzzle. Another strategy that may also lead to some of the above advantages is training twice. Performing two exercise sessions in close proximity can also bring about changes in mitochondrial biogenesis and increased fat oxidation independent of restricting carbohydrates (34).

How to implement it

The easiest way to use the low carbohydrate protocol is to train before breakfast after an overnight fast. For further benefits you would wait until 4-5hrs after your session before having any carbohydrates. If you are training in the evening you would remove carbohydrates after your session and only have a protein snack before bed.

'Train high, sleep low' is another popular protocol where a high-intensity session is performed in the evening to deplete muscle glycogen. The athlete then refrains from eating any carbohydrates post training before sleeping 'low' (without replenishing glycogen stores). The next morning the athlete performs an additional low intensity session after the overnight fast. It is important that the athlete replenishes their carbohydrate stores after this second session.

Issues with training low include a reduction in the quality of the training, an increase in perceived effort and a reduction in performance (35, 36). Caffeine and a carbohydrate mouth rinse may help with fatigue and perception of effort (37). The athlete may also increase the risk of injury and illness from overreaching, or straining their body too much (38, 37). Because of these reasons, 'train low' sessions must be carefully considered and only used sparingly.

This low carb approach is not a magic strategy and must be implemented with caution. There is a clear impairment of performance under low carb conditions, so these sessions should be carefully considered in relation to the time of day, training load and intensity. Too much too soon will only hinder performance and have a detrimental effect on the athletes training.

Training 'low' would be better suited to sessions that do not rely upon carbohydrate fuelling to begin with, including lower intensity steady state sessions below 3h and easier training days.

What about if weight loss is the goal

If weight loss is the main goal, then restricting your intake of carbohydrates can be an easy strategy to reduce overall caloric intake. However, the balance in which carbohydrate intake should be limited without it being detrimental, must be determined individually and with care (39). If you are in an energy deficit (see chapter 1), your carb to fat ratio will not be crucial (40), so use personal preference, the carbohydrate guidelines above and performance to dictate your intake of carbohydrate.

Types of carbohydrates

It is recommended that athletes consume mostly complex carbohydrates which are high in fibre (wholegrains, vegetables and fruit) for health benefits (41, 42). However, when carb needs are high, like during high intensity work out sessions, especially when training twice a day, it can be very difficult to consume sufficient amounts of complex carbs. In these cases, it is preferable to consume concentrated sources, such as juices, carb powders, carb drinks or sugary foods. This will ensure glycogen is available for before, during and after training to help with fuelling and recovery (26).

Team Sky's Carbohydrate Periodisation

Preceding the 2016 Tour De France, the cyclist Chris Froome tweeted a photo of his low carbohydrate breakfast of an avocado and a boiled egg. Many people were quick to assume that Team Sky who are arguably one of the most successful cycling team of the decade were advocates of a low carbohydrate approach. However, the team nutritionist Dr James Morton refutes this claim later explaining the real strategy behind the fuelling of the team.

Dr Morton implemented a periodised approach where carbohydrate needs were altered depending on the length and duration of the exercise session. *"Sometimes you need a lot of fuel, sometimes you don't need a lot of fuel"* (43).

During the tour, Dr Morton explains how mountainous stages required additional fuelling strategies compared to flat, less intense stages. Likewise, earlier on in the season when body composition is more of a priority, more sessions were performed under low carbohydrate conditions resulting in adaptation as well as fat loss.

This carbohydrate periodisation is a prime example of how by fuelling the work at hand enables you to train effectively, properly recover, enable the most adaptation and also see positive changes in body composition.

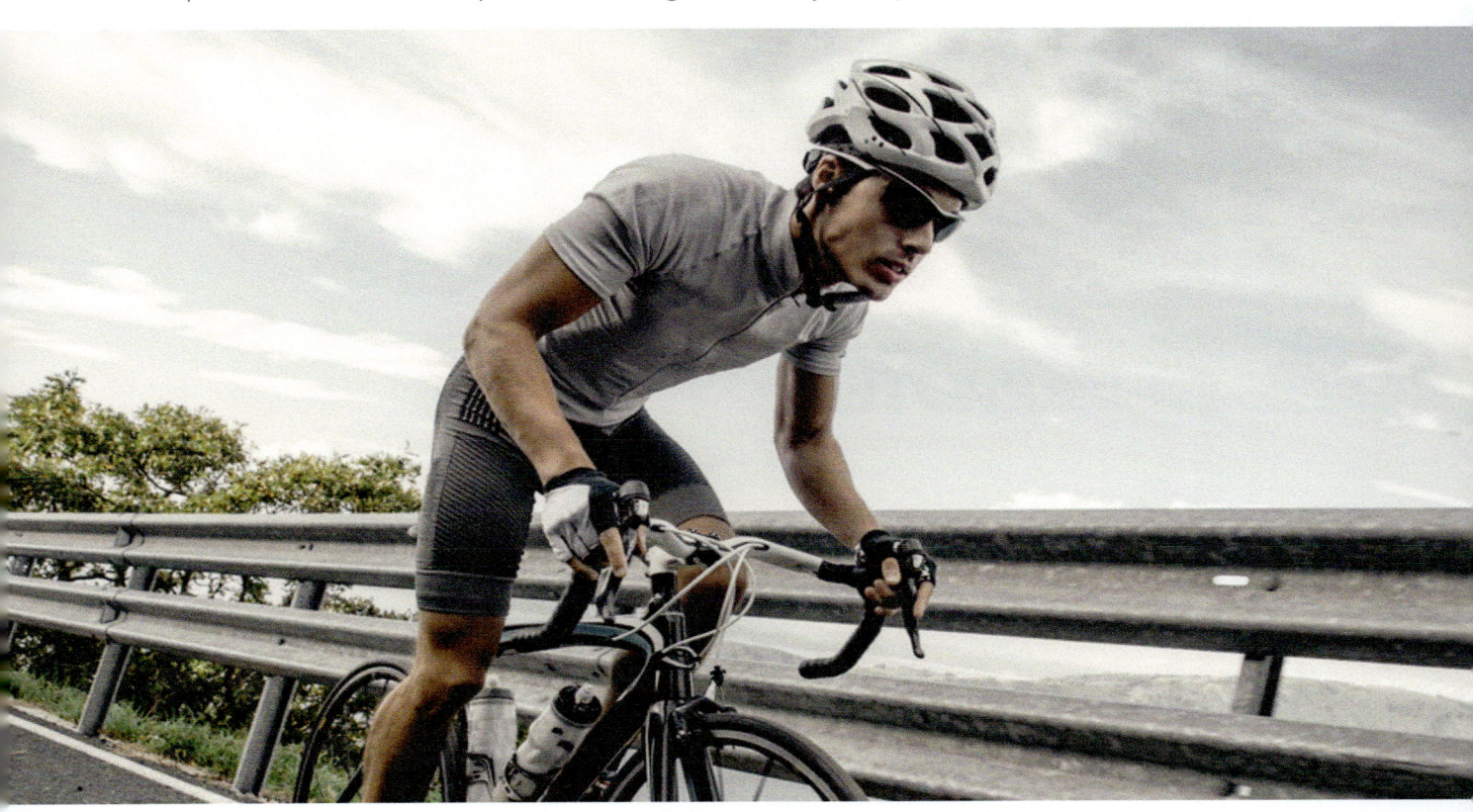

Protein

Protein is vital for repair and growth throughout the body, literally being the building block of muscle. High (relative to the average population) protein diets also consistently show improvements in body composition (44, 45, 46), strength, and hypertrophy of the muscles (size increase). Training may be the stimulus for change, but it is nutrition that facilitates the adaptation and one of the easiest, and essential ways to do this is to eat enough protein.

Protein acts as both a trigger for growth and as a substrate (the actual building block) for the formation of new muscle tissue. Both the amount of protein and the timing of protein intake are important factors for muscle size and strength. Insufficient protein intake can lead to a negative protein balance. This can, in turn, negatively impact recovery and lead to muscle breakdown. If prolonged, this causes muscle wastage, injuries and illness (44, 47, 48). So it goes without saying that sufficient protein is critical for the functional athlete.

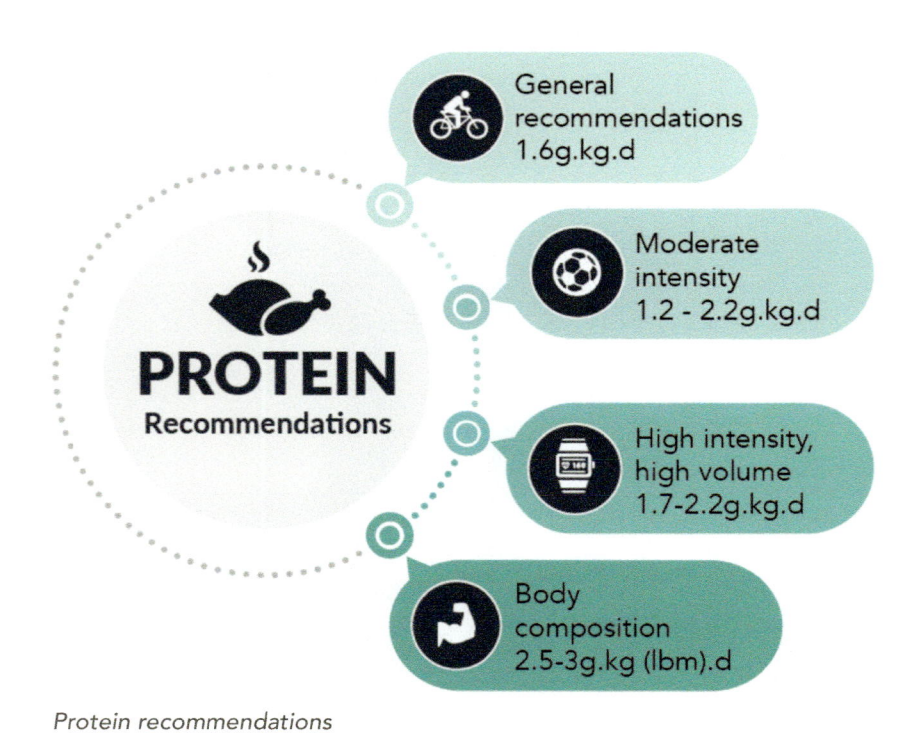

PROTEIN Recommendations

- General recommendations 1.6g.kg.d
- Moderate intensity 1.2 - 2.2g.kg.d
- High intensity, high volume 1.7-2.2g.kg.d
- Body composition 2.5-3g.kg (lbm).d

Protein recommendations

How much in total?

A good starting figure for protein consumption is around 1.6g per kg of body-weight (bw) or 2.3-2.5g per kg of Lean Body Mass (LBM) per day (10). Due to the varying nature of functional training, protein needs may differ depending on intensity of training, same as with carbohydrate. For athletes involved in moderate amounts of intense training it is recommended that they consume 1.6 –2.0g.kg.day(d) of protein, while athletes involved in high volume training should consume 1.7–2.2g.kg.d of protein. Due to the increased carbohydrate demands for endurance performance, we recommend these athletes consume around 1.4-1.8g.kg.d, which ensures proper fuelling is not being sacrificed by increasing protein intake in place of carbohydrates.

If body composition improvement is the goal, there should be an emphasis on preserving muscle mass whilst reducing fat mass which may warrant a higher intake of protein, above 2g per kg of bodyweight or 2.5-3g per kg LBM per day (44).

As muscle has a higher energy requirement than fat, calculating lean body mass enables you to work out protein requirements more precisely. This is particularly important if the athlete has a high body fat percentage.

How much per serving

To keep a positive protein balance, athletes are advised to consume 0.25-0.3g per kg of body weight (around 22-25g) interspersed throughout the day and a similar dose (0.3g.kg.bw) after exercise to maximise muscle protein synthesis (MPS). A larger bolus of protein before bed (0.6g.kg.bw) is also recommended to reduce the rate of protein breakdown (5, 26). Older individuals (53-71) are less sensitive to protein ingestion and require more (40g) per serving to optimally stimulate protein synthesis (10). The recommendations are to consume high quality sources with adequate levels of the amino acid leucine, which further promotes muscle protein synthesis (MPS) (45).

Similar to overall kcals and carbohydrates, individual factors and training schedules will dictate how much protein is necessary. An increase in volume and intensity will require a larger amount of protein (5). It's also important to be aware that if you don't match carbohydrates with energy expenditure, protein may be used to compensate for the lack of fuel, reducing its benefit for muscle growth and repair.

On the flip side, more is not always better. In strength and power sports, athletes are more likely to have excessive protein intakes (49), which could hinder performance especially if carbohydrates are being improperly replaced.

As mentioned previously, stay flexible and adjust this figure by monitoring recovery, performance, and body composition metrics.

Does the type of protein matter?

Proper daily protein intake levels should be the primary goal. However, regarding strength and size, the quality of the protein is also relevant. The quality of the protein can be determined by its amino acid content and digestion rates. Protein sources containing higher levels of the essential amino acids (those that cannot be produced by the body) are thought to be higher quality sources. Research suggests that the leucine (an amino acid) content of a food is the best determining factor when building new muscle (44). Foods which have a high leucine content include dairy, eggs, beef and fish.

Research has shown that food sources containing animal and dairy based proteins contain the highest percentage of leucine and other essential amino acids. This composition leads to greater muscle growth when compared to vegetarian proteins. However, combining vegetarian sources and adding supplemental leucine can increase the essential amino acid (EAA's) percentages and overcome any deficiencies in quality (45).

While greater doses of leucine have been shown to independently stimulate increases in protein synthesis the greatest increase comes from the combination of EAAs. So, a whole protein source like a whey shake or glass of milk will be far more effective than an amino acid isolate drink.

Protein sources high in leucine	Quantity (g)	Serving size	Protein (g)
Chicken light meat raw	100		24
Cheese/ Quark	150	0.6x Small tub	22
Whey protein isolate powder	30	1x Average serving/scoop	27
Tuna tinned in brine drained	130	1x Standard tin (180g)	32
Tofu raw regular	250	1x Cup	20

What about supplements?

Athletes should attempt to get most of their daily protein from whole foods, however larger athletes, with higher needs, may find this difficult. In these circumstances the use of supplementation (whey, soy, egg, pea, rice, vegetarian blend) can be a practical strategy to ensure you hit protein targets (45).

Fats

In addition to protein and carbohydrates, fats are the third vital macronutrient. Fats provide a good source of energy, contribute to regulating body temperature, and are crucial for the protection of internal organs.

As with protein and overall caloric intake, chronically low fat levels can inhibit fitness performance. Insufficient fat can reduce the production of testosterone thereby inhibiting the growth of new muscle (26), compromising anabolic hormone profile (key for muscle growth, strength gain and better bone mass) (50) and weakening the immune system (51). Very low-fat diets will also reduce essential fatty acids and fat-soluble vitamin intake.

For exercise

There has recently been a resurgence in promoting keto or low carb high fat (LCHF) diets for performance; however, as previously discussed, performance is inhibited if carbohydrate availability is low for various types of activities

(24), therefore it is not recommended for the functional athlete. There may be some benefit from LCHF diets in certain situations (ultra-endurance), however for high intensity activity and most strength sessions, it will only be detrimental.

A sustained low carb/high fat diet can also impair the ability to use carbohydrates for fuel by decreasing the activation of an enzyme called PDH, even when glycogen stores are repleted, this would be disastrous for any moderate to high intensity exercise or team based sports (53, 18).

So how much fat?
Fat intake should be calculated from the remainder of the athlete's daily energy needs and used as a way to complete the caloric intake, in addition to the other two major macros. Generally, it is recommended that athletes aim for around 20-30% of their daily caloric intake be from fat, and up to 50% if training volume is high (10). A healthy starting point is to keep fat around 0.8-1g per kg of bodyweight per day, where avoiding anything below 0.6g.kg.bw.

Sources
Although no fat is inherently bad (with the possible exception of trans fats), it is recommended that the majority of fat should come from unsaturated fats like oily fish, avocados, olive oil etc. If we go into details, 10–15% of daily caloric intake should be from mono-unsaturated and 10–15% from polyunsaturated fat. This ratio may help improve health markers and body composition (54). Dietary reference intakes (DRIs: Acceptable Macronutrient Distribution Ranges) recommend that you also keep saturated fat intake below 10% of your total kcals consumed.

To Sum Up.

Macronutrients.

Carbohydrates

- Carbohydrates are the primary and preferred fuel for high intensity workouts.
- Adequate carbohydrate intake is required to perform well for:

    1. High intensity interval training
    2. Moderate to intense sessions more than 2 hrs in duration
    3. High repetition weightlifting sessions
    4. For low intensity sessions and low volume weight sessions carbohydrate intake is not quite as important

- It is important to match carbohydrate needs with training volume and intensity for the given day
- You can estimate your carbohydrate needs based on goals, body weight and exercise load. Athletes should aim for around 3-7g per kg of bodyweight per day
- Be flexible and use trial and error to fine tune your daily intake
- Focus should be put on fuelling around and during sessions
- If you're training more than once per day, carbohydrates with a higher glycaemic index will be more beneficial between workouts to help with glycogen synthesis and recovery rates

Protein

- Aim for 1.6g per kg of bodyweight or 2.5g per kg of LBM per day
- Consume 0.25-0.3g per kg of body weight (around 25-40g) interspersed throughout the day and a similar dose (0.3g.kg BW) after exercise
- Aim for a higher dose (0.6g.kg.bw) before bed
- Look for sources high in EAA's and in particularly leucine

Fat

- Aim for 1g per kg of bodyweight per day or 20-30% of your caloric intake
- Avoid consuming less than 0.6g per kg of bodyweight per day
- To avoid discomfort or GI distress, keep high fat foods to a minimum around exercise
- Reduce high fat foods when glycogen synthesis and is important

The Ketogenic Diet - Something worth considering?

With its growing popularity amongst the functional fitness community, it seems only right that I address the 'Keto' elephant in the room. Although no new thing, the Ketogenic (Keto) diet has seen a significant rise in its use with it being hailed as remedy for health, weight loss and performance. So, should we be taking note?

What is the Ketogenic diet?
The Ketogenic diet is a high fat, low protein and low carbohydrate (less than 50g per day) diet. The reduction in carbohydrates forces the body to convert fat into ketone bodies that are used to fuel the muscles and brain.

Do you burn more fat?
Although forcing the body into ketosis will use more fat as fuel, this does not necessarily equate to a loss in body fat. Put simply, your body will use or 'burn' whichever food it is presented with. If you eat more fat you will use this as a fuel, whereas if you eat more carbohydrates your body will use these carbs for fuel.

Will removing carbohydrates help you lose weight?

The insulin hormone hypothesis
The main rationale behind why carbohydrates are regarded as the main factor as preventing fat loss, is the hormone insulin prevents lipolysis, which is the release of fat from your fat cells. It also increases the amount of fat taken up by these fat cells.

So, with this logic, the argument goes that cutting out carbs completely will prevent the production of insulin and enable more fatty acids to be released and used as fuel.

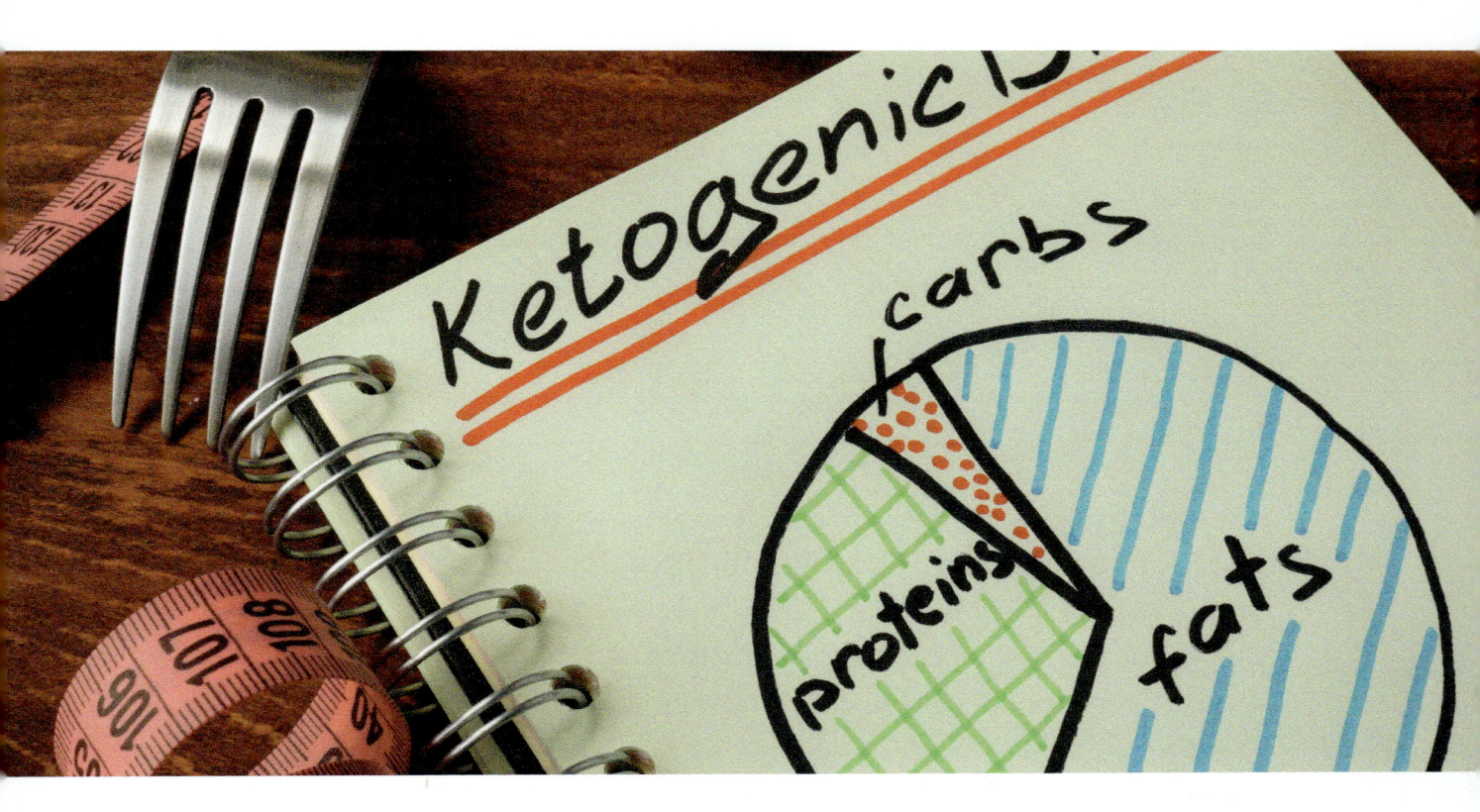

However.

1. It's not just carbohydrates that stimulate insulin
Protein is insulinemic too, which means it also spikes insulin. When combined with carbohydrates it produces a greater spike than carbohydrates alone (55), yet we know that a high (relative) protein/moderate carb diet is effective at improving body composition (56).

2. Insulin is not continually released
Insulin only has a half-life (degraded after) of around 10 minutes once released (57), so despite blocking lipolysis, this would only be for a small portion of the day.

3. Fatty acid release does not mean fat loss
Blocking insulin and enabling fatty acids to leave the cells does not necessarily equate to a loss of any body fat stores, as many of these fatty acids are taken back up into the fat cells through a process called re-esterification.

Fat flux or how fatty acids leave and enter the cells is actually a continuous process that goes on throughout the day. Even when insulin is kept low, the majority of these fatty acids will re-enter the fat cells as they're not needed (we store fat for energy after all). It's only when we have a big enough energy demand that they go through another process called beta-oxidation where they are finally used.

To use these fatty acids, you have to be in an overall energy deficit to use these fatty acids. It's the net effect that matters, not just removing carbs.

Any diet that puts you into a negative kcal balance will help you lose weight, whether it's Keto, Vegan, Paleo, Mediterranean, fasting or just eating well. When kcals and protein are matched however, there is a negligible difference in the weight you lose between a low carbohydrate and low-fat dietary approach (62). It's kcal balance which dictates fat loss, not the amount of carbohydrates.

Are there any benefits of cutting out carbs?

Yes, there are some very real practical benefits of cutting down on carbohydrates:

- *By reducing your carbohydrates, you are more likely to increase your protein intake, which in turn can help with satiety and consequently reduce your kcal intake*
- *A drop in carbohydrates will automatically reduce a lot of junk food eaten (crisps, sweets, biscuits), which will help control kcals*
- *Cutting carbohydrates will likely lead to a reduction in refined sugar and processed foods eaten. These too are foods that are more likely to promote fat gain and can make sticking to a diet more challenging*
- *Cutting out a whole food group will naturally help reduce kcals as a result of eating less*
- *Low carb or keto diets can be favourable for 'unhealthy' populations with some kind of metabolic dysfunction (poor glucose control, pre diabetic, hypertension etc) (58, 59). This is not to say low carb will cure all of these ailments, but it could be used for some therapeutic benefits*

Will it help us as functional athletes?

Put simply *'no'*. As previously discussed, for high volume, high intensity exercise that primarily uses the glycolytic pathway will require carbohydrates to perform optimally, because of the speed carbohydrates are converted to energy compared to fat. However, the use of a high fat diets may translate into a performance benefit for longer, slower endurance-based activities such as ironman and ultra-distance events (60).

There is also the danger that remaining in a low carb diet for a lengthy period of time may inhibit your ability to use and deliver carbohydrates to the muscle as fuel (61). As athletes, we want to be able to successfully switch from the use of carbohydrates and fat depending on the intensity and length of the session. This is the reason why the carbohydrate periodisation approach we recommend seems to make more sense than a solely adopting a low or high carb approach.

Is it easy to stick to?

It is generally well accepted that diets are difficult to stick to regardless of the approach. A recent research review concluded that the ketogenic diet is no different where people may start strong but have difficulty in adhering to the diet after 1-3 month (63).

To sum up

Although there may be some benefits of reducing carbohydrates, removing an entire food group, reducing fibrous and wholegrain foods that we know have enormous health benefits seems a questionable strategy at best. Even from a very practical and real-world standpoint, the prohibition of biscuits, sandwiches and beer in my eyes is quite simply a foolish proposition that I will not be recommending.

2.3 MICRONUTRIENTS

Micronutrients are the vitamins and minerals we require in small amounts to keep our bodies functioning properly. Their functions range from things such as energy and bone health to immunity and recovery. In most cases, provided you are eating a well-balanced diet, additional micronutrient supplementation should not be required and will not lead to an improvement in performance or health.

For the majority of athletes who consume a nutrient rich and well-balanced diet, will have all their vitamin and mineral needs fulfilled by their nutrition. There will be no need for additional supplementation. In fact, supplementing above the RDA's (recommended daily allowance) may result in negative consequences.

There are some exceptions where precautions should be taken to ensure adequate micronutrient availability. Athletes who restrict energy intake, remove whole food groups, undertake severe weight loss strategies or are vegetarian/vegan can put themselves at risk of deficiency of certain vitamins and minerals (64, 5).

So which ones?

Vitamin D
Vitamin D is synthesized in the skin when it is exposed to sunlight. It helps calcium absorption and is key for maintaining good bone health (65). A recent surge in research has also highlighted the correlation between sufficient vitamin D and injury prevention, muscular function, muscle strength (66), reduced

inflammation, and decreased risk of illness (5).

Who needs it? Anyone who lives at latitudes beneath the 35th parallel is less likely to get vitamin D from the sun. If you have a darker complexion or avoid the sun you might be at risk of deficiency (67).

Recent research suggests that the current DRI (dietary reference intake) of 10 µg/d (400 IU/d) (68) may be difficult to reach without supplementation. There is currently not enough empirical evidence to claim that vitamin D is an ergogenic aid or that it directly improves performance; however, if you live in the colder regions or rarely see sunshine, then supplementation maybe worthwhile.

High dose antioxidants

High doses of vitamins E and C have been shown to reduce oxidative stress caused by exercise. However, although this may reduce pain and muscle damage, this oxidative stress is what leads to adaptation (strength gains), so high dose antioxidants can negatively affect performance if used too often (69). This is the reason why you should only use additional high dose antioxidants during competition or during an intense period of training when recovery is particularly important. This will help keep acute damage to a minimum.

Iron

Iron is required by the body for transporting oxygen from the lungs to the muscle. Across all areas of functional fitness, oxygen carrying capacity is obviously vital, not just for endurance, but also for cognitive function and immunity (70). Inadequate iron can impair and limit work capacity as well as muscle function, health, and cognitive performance (64, 71). Iron deficiency is important to consider for those participating in high intensity or endurance activities not only because of the increased oxygen demands but also because high impact sports can cause hemolysis (the destruction of red blood cells) by repetitive prolonged damage. Vegetarians on the whole are more likely to have an iron-poor diet and women tend to be at a greater risk for deficiency due to menstrual blood loss and an increased likelihood of restricted eating (72).

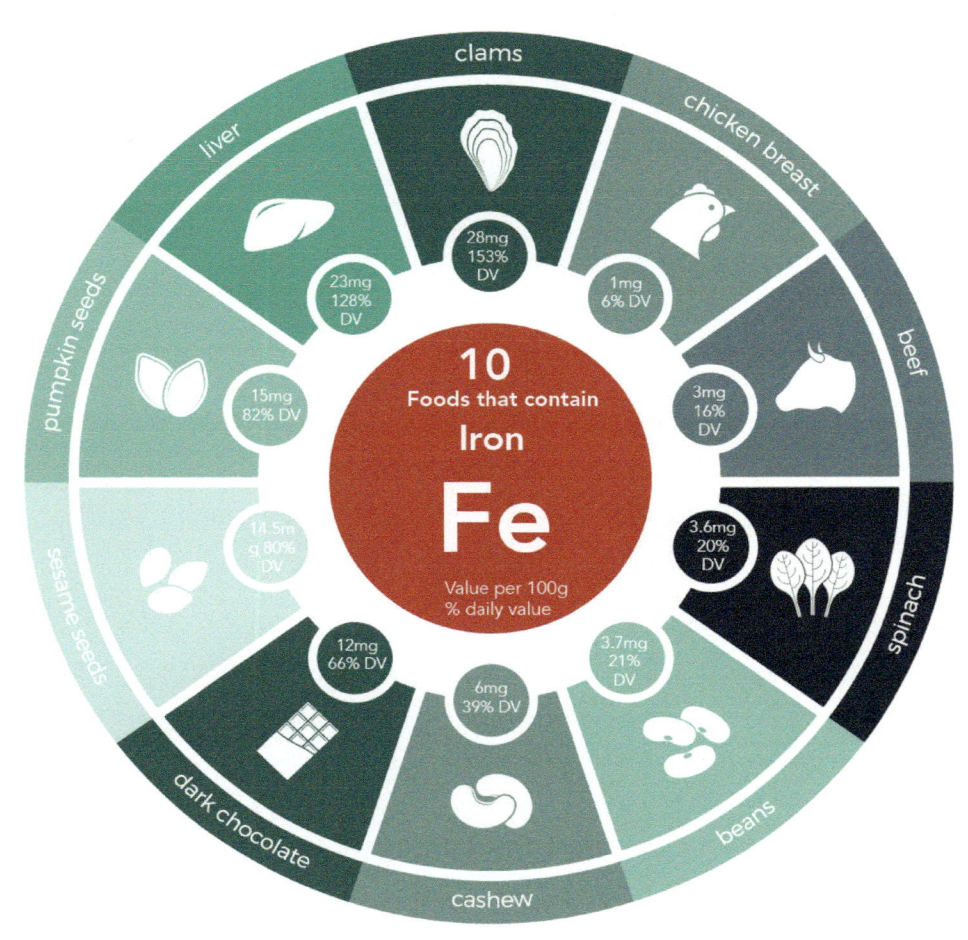

Iron sources

Populations at risk like those mentioned should aim for an intake greater than the NHS recommended daily amount (14.8mg for women and >8mg for men). You can achieve that by following these simple guidelines:

- *Eat foods rich in heme iron at least 4 times a week (e.g. liver or red meat)*
- *Include non-heme iron food sources (e.g., dried fruit, legumes, and green leafy vegetables)*
- *Combine non heme-iron foods with meat or vitamin C-rich food (like orange juice) to increase iron absorption*
- *Avoid drinking tea with meals*
- *Avoid supplementation post exercise as absorption is reduced (60)*

Calcium

Since calcium is responsible for growth, muscle contractions, and bone repair, it is important that athletes get enough in their diets. A deficiency can lead to decreased bone density and an increased likelihood of stress fractures and osteoporosis. Issues arise from low energy availability (not eating enough or excessive exercise), eating disorders, and avoidance of dairy or calcium rich foods (5). This further highlight that if you are eating a balanced diet comprised of dairy, fish (with bones!), and dark vegetables, then you should comfortably attain the RDA of 1000mg per day and supplementation should not be necessary.

Zinc

Zinc is another micronutrient found in meat, eggs and legumes that, if deficient, can impact the health of individuals. For athletes who partake in prolonged intense exercise, zinc supplementation (25mg/d) can help support immune function and reduce the risk of upper respiratory tract infections (73, 74).

To sum up

A well-balanced, nutrient rich diet typically supplies all the necessary micronutrients without the need for supplementation. However, due to possible heavy demands of the functional athlete, supplementation may sometimes be warranted. It would be wise to be tested for Vitamin D and iron and then make an informed decision based on training requirements and performance. Look out for common symptoms associated with a deficiency (are you getting injured frequently, struggling to recover, or consistently lacking energy?) and in the meantime, make a concerted effort to eat a nutrient dense, varied diet.

3

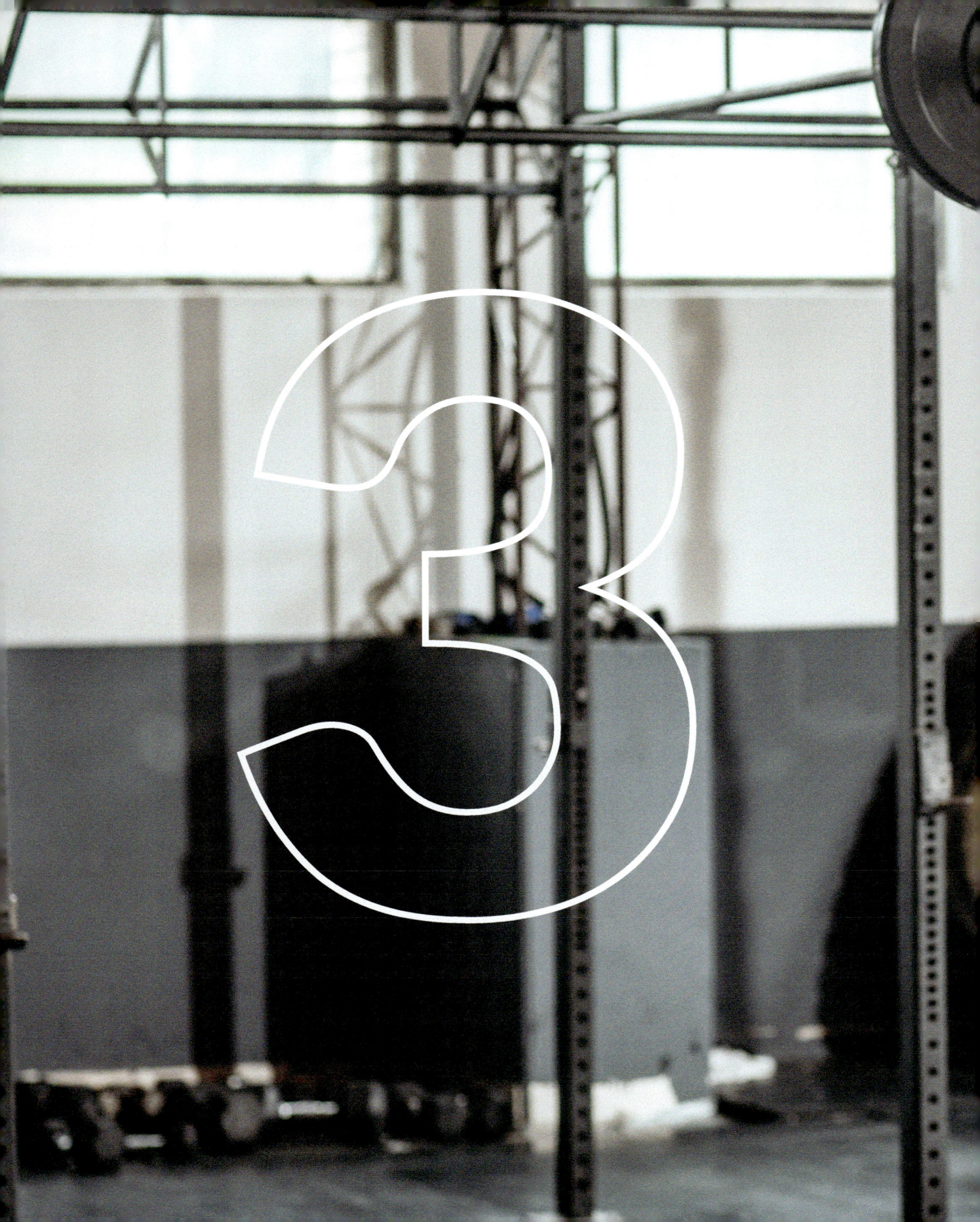

CHAPTER THREE

FUELLING YOUR TRAINING

3.1 FUELLING YOUR TRAINING

Although your overall diet will have the biggest impact on performance, understanding workout nutrition correctly will help fuel and support your individual training sessions. Adjusting your intake around your workout schedule will help mitigate fatigue, facilitate maximum adaptation to training and help recovery (1, 2). For this we must consider carbohydrate availability, hydration/electrolyte balance, and protein intake.

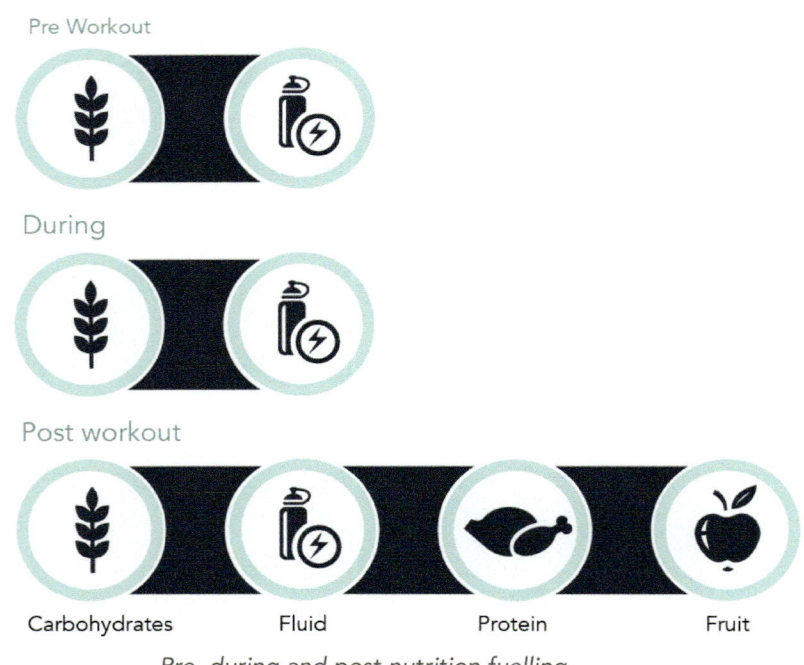

Pre Workout

During

Post workout

Carbohydrates   Fluid   Protein   Fruit

Pre, during and post nutrition fuelling

Carbohydrates

The amount of carbohydrates you require for each session will depend on the duration, intensity and type of exercise. As previously discussed in the carbohydrates section, workout plans that include HIT training, prolonged moderate to intense endurance workouts that are less than 2hrs and for weights sessions with high repetitions, adequate carbohydrates are required.

Fuelling yourself with carbohydrates before these types of sessions will have a more positive effect on performance as opposed to training fasted (training without eating beforehand) (3, 4). As your sessions increase in length, having more carbohydrate available to use as fuel will increase performance. On the other hand, low availability of carbohydrate will lead to fatigue, impaired skill, and increased perceived exertion (5, 6). As workouts extend past 20 minutes, the body relies more on glycogen availability (stored carbohydrates). A clear link exists between glycogen depletion and exercise performance.

At a high intensity, glycogen depletion is more rapid in fast twitch muscle fibres compared to slow twitch fibres (7). This means that even though glycogen stores in all muscle types, on average, may be only moderately depleted, your fast twitch fibres may be completely depleted, decreasing your ability to perform at high intensity.

For this reason, it is important to top off glycogen levels before training and maintain blood glucose during longer sessions.

What about low rep power and strength training?

As discussed in the previous chapter, lower volume and shorter resistance training sessions will not deplete stored carbohydrates like endurance training does. A specific pre-workout nutrition protocol is unlikely to bring about any performance benefits for low rep power and strength training, if they are not very long. Focus instead on your collective nutrition for the day.

PRE-WORKOUT NUTRITION

Carbohydrates

Consuming carbohydrates before exercise will replenish glycogen in the liver, which will be depleted due to the overnight fast. This will ensure that there is blood glucose available during your first workout. For workouts longer than 60mins of moderate or intense exercise aim for an intake of around 1-1.4g.kg of bodyweight of carbohydrates (8, 9). For shorter workouts and strength sessions this amount may not be necessary. However, we still recommend a bolus of carbohydrates before you train, despite your overall carbohydrate numbers throughout the day being more important.

Timing

It takes roughly 4hrs for carbohydrates to be stored in the muscles and liver as glycogen, so eating around 4-6 hours before your workout is ideal. You may also consider a smaller snack 30 minutes prior to your first workout of the day to help increase carbohydrate availability in your blood. Take care to avoid foods high in fibre or fats before workouts, to minimize chances of gastrointestinal problems.

The size of your meal will depend on how soon you eat before exercising. The less time you have until your exercise routine, the less quantity you should eat. If you have more time until exercise, its ok to have a larger meal. If you are training early in the day and you do not have enough time to digest a larger meal, you can choose liquid or semi liquid nutrition to help speed up digestion rates. You can also have a larger meal the night before, to stock up for the morning. Be aware that eating 60 minutes or less before your workout may result in feeling more fatigued than not having eaten at all. This comes from a drop in blood glucose levels caused by a rise in insulin (10). Therefore, the timing and type of food should be based on individual preferences and daily schedule. Practise, experiment and find a setup that suits you.

Type

There is a lot of debate about whether low GI or high GI carbohydrates are more beneficial for performance. Most of the research supports the notion that lower GI carbohydrates sustains exercise for longer than higher GI foods because they provide a continuous source of energy for longer (11, 12). This may also be due to the body's use of fat as fuel for the start of the workout, sparing glycogen for later in the workout. Your schedule will dictate which is more practical. If you don't have much time before your session or competition, quickly digesting carbohydrates will still provide an immediate energy supply.

Sources	Quantity	Calories	Carbs (g)
Lucozade	1 bottle	266	55
Gatorade	1 bottle	130	35
Carbs powder	50g	185	50
Fruit juice	250ml	120	30

Hydration

Drinking enough water is critical for health and performance. Dehydration hinders the body's ability to remove heat. This can lead to:

Strain on the cardiovascular system
Reduced fluid absorption
Risk of heat illness

A 2% drop in body weight due to water loss can significantly hinder cognitive function and exercise capacity. A 3-5% drop in water weight impacts high intensity performance and sport-specific skills (8).

Although there are individual differences among athletes, it is recommended that you drink around 5-10 ml.kg.bw (ref p.34) of water 2-4 hours before exercise. An easy method to help ensure you are hydrated before exercise is to check your urine colour against the hydration chart. This can be found in your progress tracker in the resource section. The darker your urine is, the more dehydrated you are. A light 'like lemonade' colour helps indicate good hydration.

DURING EXERCISE

Carbohydrates

For workouts that last less than 90 minutes, intra-workout carbohydrates are not necessary. However, during longer and more intense sessions, glycogen depletion may require additional carbs during the workout to help with glucose availability in the muscle. The athlete should look for foods, drinks, and gels that are easily digested and won't cause any stomach complaints (1, 5, 13). For sessions lasting longer than 90 mins at a high intensity (> 70% VO2Max) aim to consume 30-60g of carbohydrates per hour in a 6–8% carbohydrate-electrolyte solution (around 200ml) every 15 minutes.

Combining your carbohydrates

Research shows that combining different types of carbohydrates (glucose and fructose) enables you to ingest more (90g/hr) compared to using one source (14). This is because glucose and fructose use different transporters for absorption. For events lasting longer than 3 hrs, it is recommended to combine these two carbohydrates to help increase absorption rates, which can lead to improvements in performance (15).

Athletes should aim to consume a 2:1 glucose: fructose ratio, however many sports drinks already have that ratio.

More than just a fuel

Carbohydrates not only affect the level of energy available to you, but also the skill level at which activity is performed *"Carbohydrate intake has been associated with significantly better maintenance of whole-body motor skills and mood state, and reduced perception of exertion, fatigue and force production"* (16). With glucose being the preferred fuel for the brain, a drop in available carbohydrate levels can lead to 'mental fatigue' which is not ideal for any skill-based type of activities or sports. When this happens, perceived exertion may be alleviated though intra-workout carbs or even a carbohydrate mouth rinse (rinsing a carbohydrate solution around the mouth and spitting it out) (17).

Hydration

During training, athletes should try and replace fluid lost by sweating with around 0.4-0.8 l/hr of either water or an electrolyte sports drink depending on the carbohydrate needs. Colder drinks help to keep core temperature down. There will be individual differences, so stay flexible and increase your fluid intake to compensate for increased sweating. It's better to err on the upper side with fluids, than risk dehydration.

AFTER YOU EXERCISE - THE FOUR R'S OF RECOVERY

Post exercise, the athlete needs to consider 4 key elements:
- *Refuel – Replenishment of carbohydrate stores (glycogen)*
- *Rehydrate – Replacement of lost fluid and electrolytes*
- *Repair – Rebuilding and regeneration of muscle tissue*
- *Revitalise – bolster recovery of the body's immune defence*

4 R's of Recovery

| Refuel | Rehydrate | Repair | Revitalise |

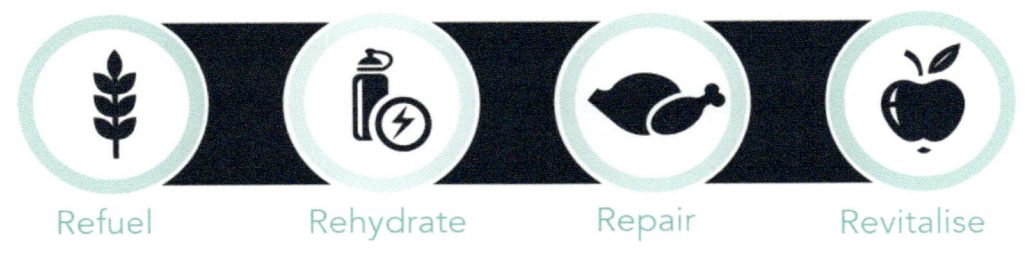

4 r's of recovery

Refuel

Exercise depletes carbohydrate stores, so replenishing them after your session should be your primary goal. After training, aim to consume ≈1g of carbohydrate per kg of body weight within 30 mins as your muscles are more readily open to store these carbs at this point. This has been shown to speed up glycogen synthesis and improve recovery (18, 19). Waiting more than two hours before you eat can lower the rate of glycogen synthesis by up to 50% (20). Higher GI carbs (more sugary foods) are better at replenishing glycogen stores, but if you have over 8 hours until your next session, it will not matter whether you eat higher GI or lower GI carbs since your body will have plenty of time to absorb and store these foods.

Rehydrate

After training you should try to achieve adequate hydration by consuming slightly more than body weight lost during exercise. So, for every 1kg lost in weight, drink around 1.25l of fluid (13). Also use urine colour to help gauge rehydration. You can also use a hydration chart to understand your fluid needs for different sessions.

A note on salt

A loss of sodium through heavy sweating can potentially lead to hyponatremia (a drop in sodium levels in the blood) and electrolyte imbalances, which will impair performance and can also be dangerous. Aim to consume foods and liquids that contain sodium to help maintain fluid balance such as electrolyte powders/tablets/sachets or sports drinks.

Repair

Even though both exercise and protein intake initiates protein synthesis independently, combining the two will elicit a greater adaptation effect. Exercising makes the muscles receptive to amino acids by increasing amino acid transporters on the muscle cell wall. As Kevin Currell (20) put it, *"Think of it as the muscle opening more doors after exercise to allow amino acids to enter the muscle."*

For this reason, it is recommended that you consume 0.3g.kg.bw (ref p.34) of protein after training, however research suggests that overall protein intake in a day outweighs the importance of pre, intra and post workout feeding alone (21). The sensitivity of the muscle lasts for up to 24hrs, so provided you consume an adequate amount of protein over the course of the day, it should not make a significant difference. It is still safe to assume that to support growth and recovery you should consume protein when you can after training. However, don't feel the need to run to the changing room to grab your shake immediately after your workout!

Revitalise

Due to the demands of training, increased exposure to pathogens (breathing hard, wounds), increased stress and under-nutrition can leave athletes at risk of illness in the post exercise period. Anti-oxidant rich foods have also been shown to help improve recovery and reduce muscle soreness (22). For this reason, we recommend including a variety of antioxidant rich foods such as fruit, vegetables, fish, nuts, olive oil and wholegrains in the post exercise period diet.

The type of session

The duration and intensity of the session will dictate what recovery strategies to follow. High volume, intense training and where two sessions are performed within 8hrs then the 4 R's are more important to follow. For lighter sessions then the next meal after training will be enough for recovery.

We are all different

There is no 'perfect' setup. Individual differences will play a big part in what works for you. Therefore, refining your diet before an event or competition is vital if you want to perform your best.

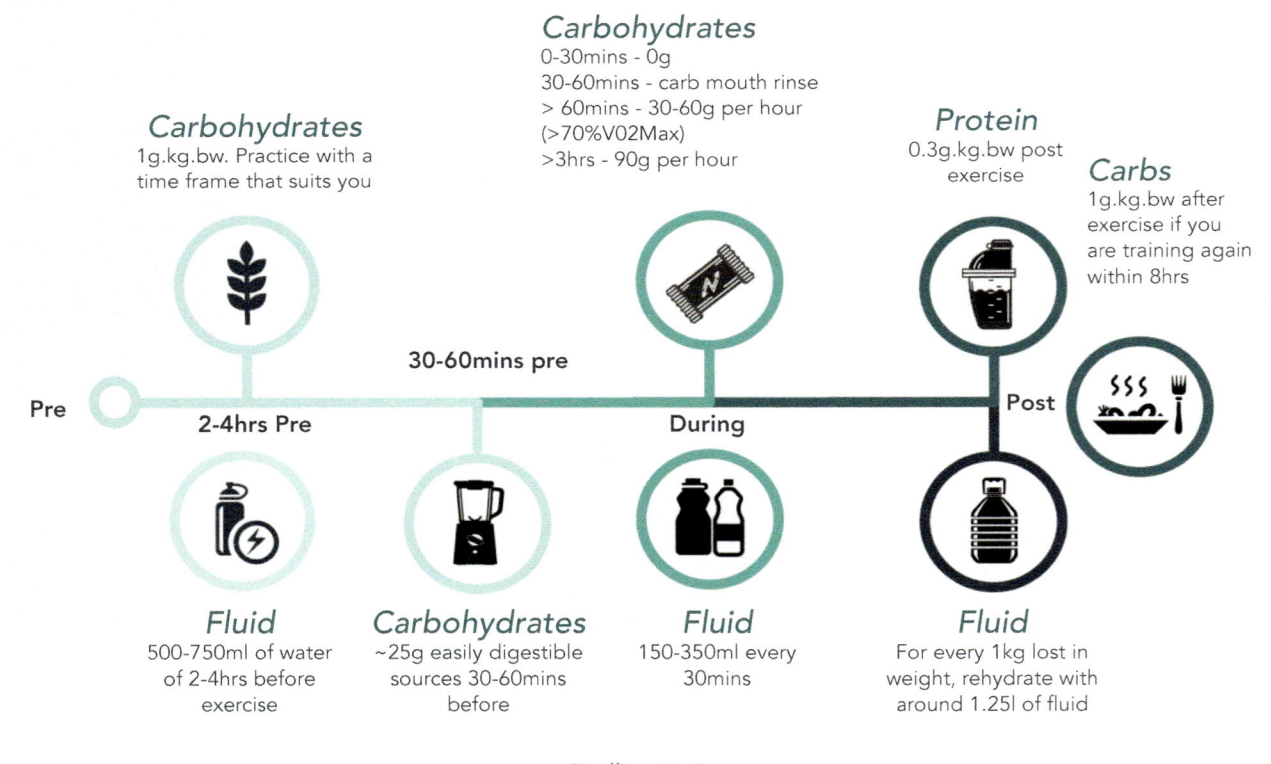

Pre

Carbohydrates
1g.kg.bw. Practice with a time frame that suits you

Fluid
500-750ml of water of 2-4hrs before exercise

2-4hrs Pre

Carbohydrates
~25g easily digestible sources 30-60mins before

30-60mins pre

During

Carbohydrates
0-30mins - 0g
30-60mins - carb mouth rinse
> 60mins - 30-60g per hour (>70%VO2Max)
>3hrs - 90g per hour

Fluid
150-350ml every 30mins

Post

Protein
0.3g.kg.bw post exercise

Carbs
1g.kg.bw after exercise if you are training again within 8hrs

Fluid
For every 1kg lost in weight, rehydrate with around 1.25l of fluid

Fuelling timing

64 FUELLING THE FUNCTIONAL ATHLETE

To Sum Up.

Fuelling Your Training

Carbohydrates

- Maintain enough carbohydrates based on the type of exercise, length of sessions and your preference
- To ensure adequate glycogen for your training, your pre-training meal should have around 1-1.4g per kg of carbohydrates
- Intra-workout carbohydrates should not be necessary for workouts less than 45mins, however, drinks, gels, bars, or even a mouth rinse can help with perceived exertion and motor control
- For sessions lasting beyond 90 mins at a high intensity (>70% VO2Max) aim to consume 30-60g of carbohydrates/hour in a 6–8% carbohydrate-electrolyte solution (around 200ml) every 15 minutes
- Aim to consume 1g per kg of body weight within the first 2hrs after exercise to replenish glycogen
- Choose high GI carbs if you plan to exercise again within the next 8hrs
- Practice with timings and foods to suit your preference and comfort
- In general, reduce high fibre foods and fats before you exercise

Protein

- Aim for 0.5g per kg of protein after you exercise
- Your focus should be on overall protein intake for the day and regular feedings rather than eating around exercise

Hydration

- Drink 5-10ml per kg of bodyweight 2-4 hours before exercise
- Try and replace fluid lost by sweating by aiming for 0.4-0.8l/h
- After training, consume slightly more water than weight lost (for every 1kg lost in weight, rehydrate with around 1.25l of fluid)

SAMPLE STRATEGY

Pre-workout

Why	Top up glycogen stores and ensure hydration	
When	2-4hours pre-workout	30-60mins pre-workout
What	Balanced solid meal of carbs and protein. Choose a carb source which you prefer and try and build up a pattern of what food types work best for you. This is the same for protein, don't get hung up about which foods are best. Keep fat relatively low.	Liquid or semi-liquid carbs for easy digestion.
Carbs	1-1.4g per kg of bodyweight	~ 25g (play with quantities to suit you)
	Example 70kg athlete. 70 x 1 and 1.4 = between 70 and 98g of carbs Example 90kg athlete. 90 x 1.2 = between 90 and 126g of carbs	

Protein	Optional 0.3g per kg of bodyweight
	Example 70kg athlete. 70 x 0.3 = 21g of protein Example 90kg athlete. 90 x 0.3 = 27g of protein
Example	- Oats, fruit, and whey protein - Peanut butter and jam bagel - Jacket potato with tuna - Chicken and pasta salad - Fish, vegetables, and potatoes	- Cereal bar - Banana - Smoothie - Dried fruit - Yoghurt - Energy drink - Gatorade/Powerade - Carbohydrate powder - Peanut butter and jam sandwich - Energy bar/shake
Fluid	Drink between 500-750ml of water of 2-4hrs before your first event

Intra workout - Sessions ≥ 60 mins

Why	Replace fluid loss. Maintain blood sugar levels
When	Every 30-60mins
What	High GI (sugary) foods to speed up glycogen replenishment
Carbs	0-30mins session - zero 30-60mins session - carbohydrate mouth rinse > 60mins session - 30-60g per hour (>70%VO2Max) >3hrs - 90g per hour* - This will vary between individuals
Fluid	Try not to use thirst as an indication of hydration, instead form a set pattern of drinking regularly. When it's very hot, drink as much as you can tolerate with electrolytes. You're looking for around 150-350ml every 30mins.
Examples:	Carbohydrate drink (SIS) Lucozade/Powerade (practise with these first) - A 6-8% isotonic drink is recommended Jaffa cakes/rice crispy squares Flapjack/cereal/granola bars Jelly babies Maltloaf Dried fruit

Post Workout

Why	Recover with protein, replenish glycogen, rehydrate
When	Immediately after workout
What	A combination of moderate to high GI carbs, protein and fat.
Carbs	1-1.2g per kg of bodyweight for each meal if you're training again within 8hrs
Protein	0.3g per kg of bodyweight
Fluid	For every 1kg lost in weight, rehydrate with around 1.25l of fluid. This may alter depending on the type of workout/session, which is why it's recommended to use a hydration chart.
Examples	Any large carbohydrate meal Pasta and tomato sauce with chicken or Bolognese Tuna and jacket potatoes, salad and fruit Chilli con carne with rice Pizza with added chicken on top Stir fry beef with noodles Ensure you have plenty of sodium (salt) to replenish what is lost through sweat. This is when certain fast foods can be good options! Avoid alcohol during this time

4

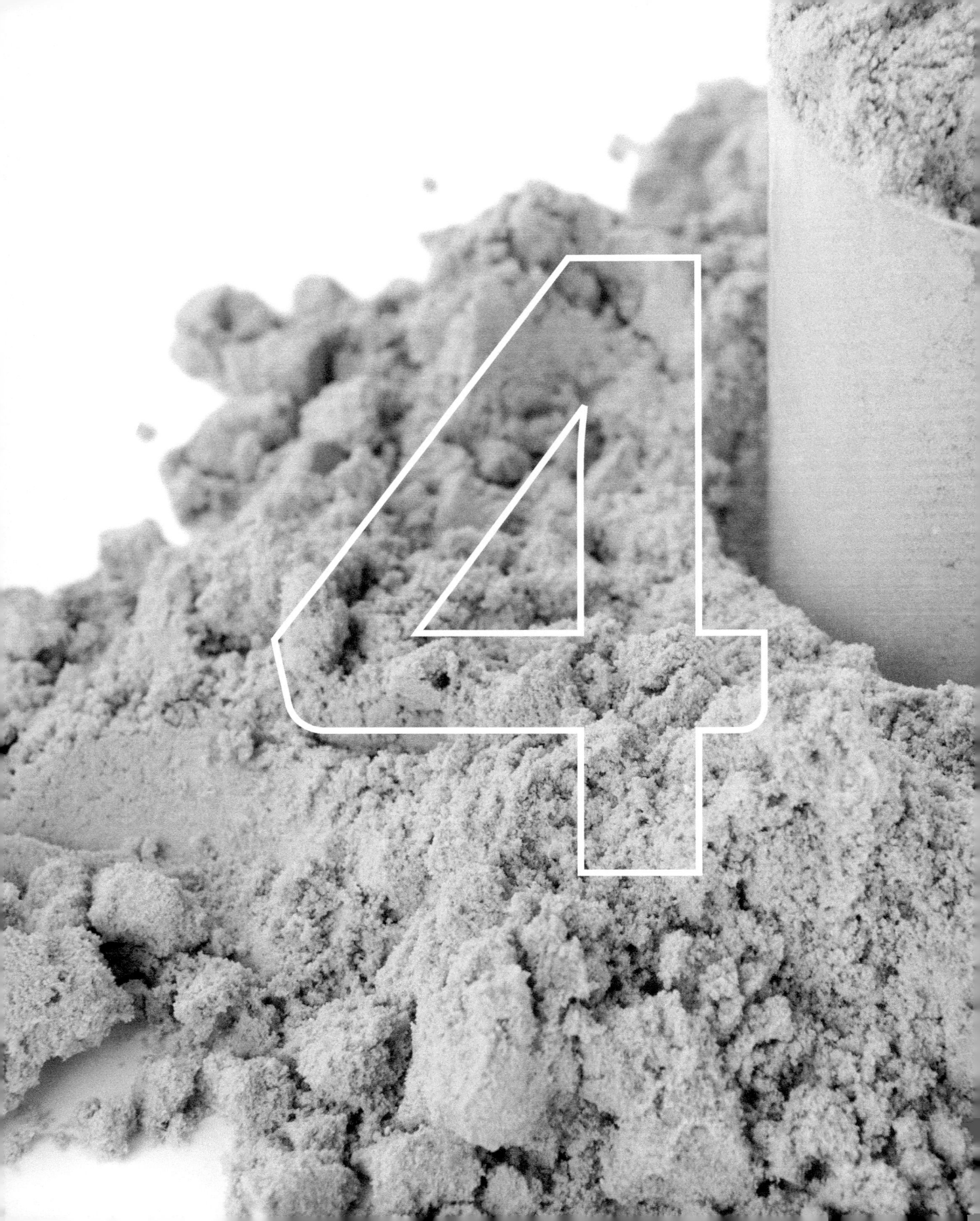

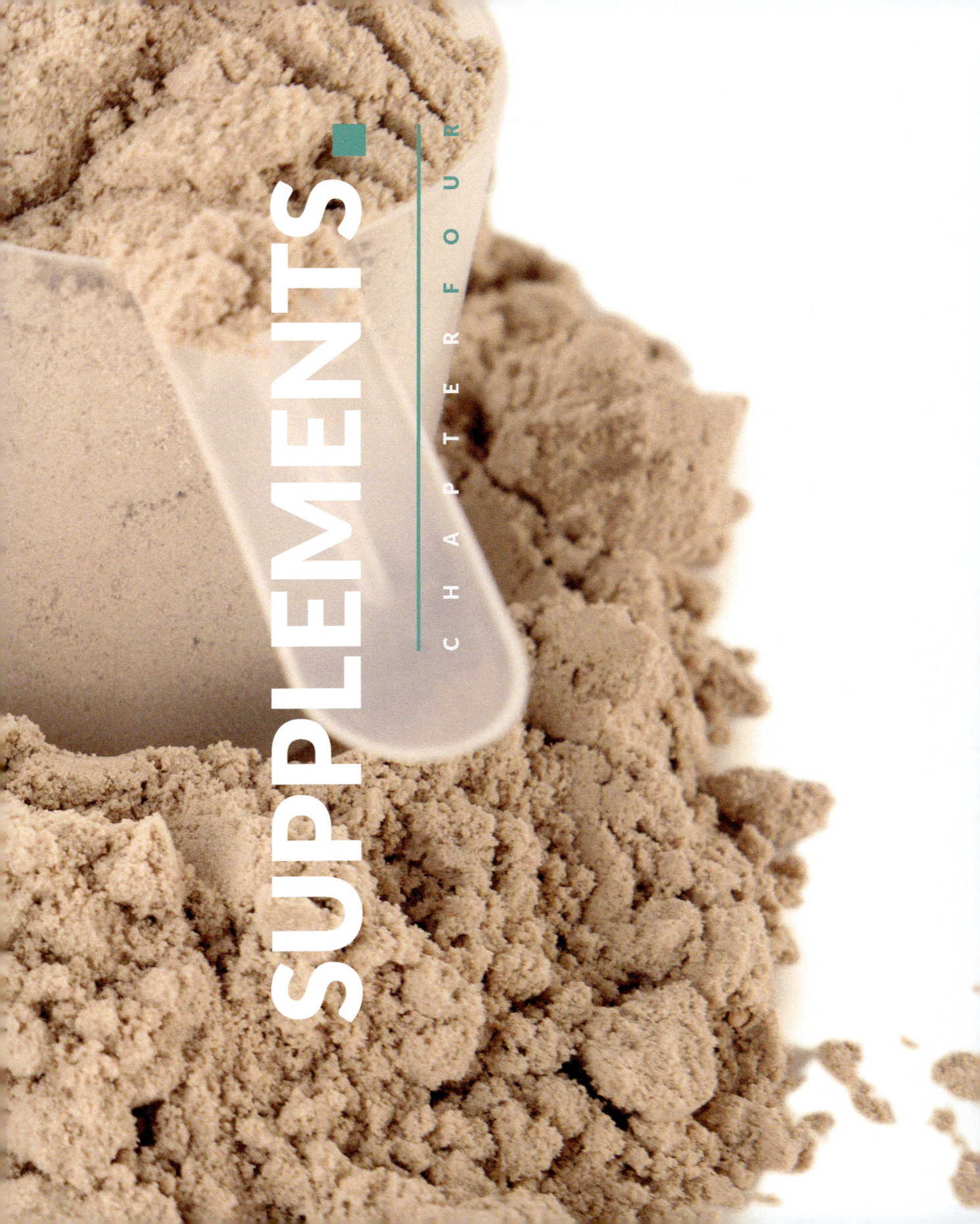

SUPPLEMENTS

CHAPTER FOUR

4.1 SUPPLEMENTS

As the name suggests, supplements should only supplement an already healthy diet. Amounts, types of food, and nutrient timing should be your primary focus. However, supplements which can help with nutrient deficiencies, training adaptation, improving performance and recovery should be considered.

This is not an exhaustive list, nor does it account for individual needs. It gives an overview of the supplements that may contribute to a positive effect on both health and performance. Remember to consult a doctor before taking any supplements, especially if you are already taking prescription medication.

Protein

For some larger athletes, it can be difficult to hit protein targets from food alone. Therefore, protein powder is a useful addition to bolster protein intake. It is also convenient, cost effective and most are high in the amino acid leucine. If you're lactose intolerant then consider an egg, soy or vegan blend, which have also been shown to increase protein synthesis that can lead to an increase in muscle mass.

Meal replacements shakes, ready to drink supplements and protein bars can also provide an easy cost effective and convenient way to help boost nutrient needs and help achieve protein and kcal goals. For athletes working long hours or on the move then these types of products can be a useful addition to the diet.

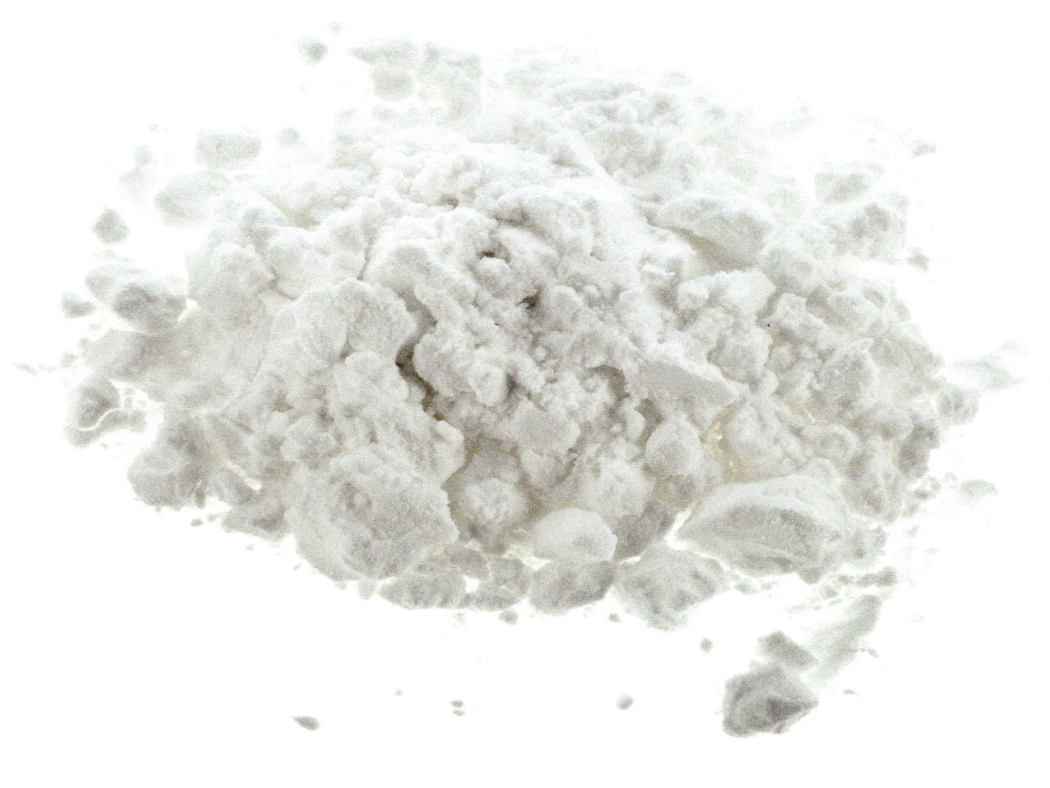

Creatine

In terms of increasing high-intensity work capacity and lean body mass during training, creatine monohydrate is the most effective performance enhancing supplement currently available to athletes (1). Creatine has been shown to increase strength, power, and fat free mass (2, 3). It may also benefit high intensity exercise and even endurance training (4), making it a perfect fit for athletes participating in power and endurance-based sports. Results vary depending on the individual, so make sure that you pay attention to how you feel and determine whether the supplement is beneficial for you. It may cause weight gain and water retention that could make your longer workouts and gymnastic movements harder. If this is the case, try to load your creatine after your training or remove it from your diet leading up to your event. Creatine has about a 4-6 week washout period (5), so you could come off creatine if you worry about water retention.

How do you take it?
The quickest way to increase your stores of creatine is to load (start) at 0.3g.kg.bw per day for approximately a week and then follow by taking 3-5g per day. You can also gradually saturate your stores by loading with 3-5g per day for 3-4 weeks.

Beta alanine

Beta alanine is a non-essential amino acid needed for the synthesis of carnosine, a compound that acts as a buffer to muscle acidosis during high exercise and helps reduce fatigue (6). Beta alanine supplementation has been shown to increase concentration and improve performance in several high intensity activities lasting 1-4 minutes and even up to 9 minutes (7). This makes it a great addition for athletes.

How to take it?
Like creatine, beta alanine requires continuous supplementation to have any effect (1g in your pre-workout shake will not do much good). A loading period of 4-6g per day for 4-6 weeks is needed to saturate carnosine stores in order to see performance benefits.

Do you struggle with the tingly sensation? Then divide your dose over the course of the day and ingest with each meal.

Caffeine

Caffeine tablets are an effective way to boost endurance performance and reduce fatigue. Caffeine has been shown to improve performance in several different activities, including endurance and high-intensity exercise (8, 9, 10, 11). Although the literature is divided on the direct impact of caffeine on maximal strength, its ability to improve mood and reduce pain reception makes it a worthwhile addition before any session.

Caffeine is more effective when consumed in an anhydrous state as opposed to liquid forms like coffee (12).

How to take it?
Caffeine improves performance when consumed at a dosage of 3-6mg.kg.bw 30-60 mins before training. This equates to around 200-600 mg. Most caffeine tablets contain 200mg. There are no additional benefits associated with a higher dose and there could be adverse effects. People also have different tolerances for caffeine, if you are sensitive to it be aware that it may affect your sleep.

Sodium Bicarbonate

Like beta alanine, sodium bicarbonate also acts as a buffering agent that prevents acidosis of the muscle, providing a potential benefit for high-intensity exercise performance. The literature suggests that sodium bicarbonate supplementation is particularly effective for exercise lasting between 1-3 minutes and potentially team sports that require short bursts of energy (13).

How to take it
It is recommended to take 0.3g.kg.bw 1-2hrs prior to exercise. One of the potential pitfalls with sodium bicarbonate is gastrointestinal distress (needing the toilet!), therefore it is advised that you practice taking smaller doses or split the dose and consume with meals prior to any exercise.

Concentrated Beetroot Juice

Eating a lot of beetroot (or foods high in nitrate) can help increase plasma nitrite, which in turn can increase nitric oxide in the body. This increase in nitric oxide can reduce the amount of oxygen needed for moderate intensity exercise and enables you to perform longer during this type of activity.

Concentrated beetroot juices have been developed as a way for athletes to gain the benefits of beetroot. The literature suggests that continuous (long term) and acute (immediately pre-workout) dosing of these types of supplements may improve your work capacity and endurance performance (13).

The evidence for the effect of these supplements on overall performance is slim and more work needs to be done in studying the results among trained athletes across different populations and activities. Currently, the literature only suggests a small incremental improvement in performance and one paper showed nitrate supplementation did not improve overall CrossFit® performance, only the time it took to complete 2000m of rowing (14).

There is also some literature which supports the health benefits of daily consumption of beetroot juice in older populations including improved blood flow and reduced blood pressure (15).

Although it may not provide a huge performance benefit, for competitions or if cost is not a problem then a shot of concentrated beetroot juice may be a worthwhile addition to the diet. Alternatively, the introduction of foods containing nitrate such as beetroot.

How to take it
Look to include high nitrate containing foods such as beetroot, spinach and rocket as part of your diet. You can also consume a concentrated shot of nitrate (310–560 mg) 2-3hrs prior to training or competing (16).

High dose antioxidants

As previously mentioned, high doses of vitamins E and C have been shown to reduce oxidative stress caused by exercise. Although this may reduce pain and muscle damage, this oxidative stress is what leads to adaptation (strength gains), so high dose antioxidants can have a negative effect on performance if used too frequently (17). This is the reason why you should only use additional high dose antioxidants during competitions or during intense training blocks when recovery is particularly important.

Citrulline Malate

Citrulline malate may be used to reduce the feeling of fatigue, increase ATP (energy) production and arginine levels that in turn increases nitric oxide. This may support anaerobic activities and sports with short rest periods (18, 19). Although the literature is promising, it is still not strong enough to guarantee a noticeable improvement.

Performance Box

Performance Box is a supplement pack designed for functional fitness athletes. Each box contains 4 weeks supply of supplements that help to improve strength, speed, lean mass, power, work capacity and recovery. To find out more visit **www.boxnutrition.co.uk/shop**

Supplement timeline

Sodium Bicarbonate
0.2-0.4g per kg of bodyweight, 1-2.5hrs pre-workout

Nitrate
6.4-12.8mg per kg of bodyweight 2-3 pre-workout

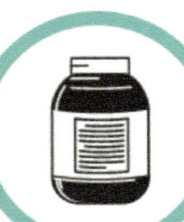

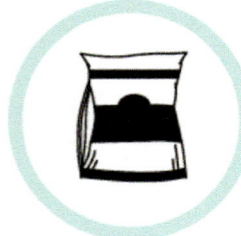

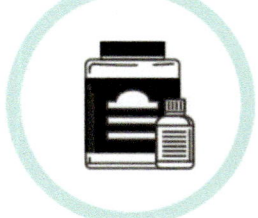

Beta alanine
4g per day for 28 days

Creatine
0.3g per kg of bodyweight for 7 days followed by 3-5g per day thereafter

4 weeks — 1 weeks — 3hrs — 2hrs

Carbohydrates

30-60g per hour for workouts > 60mins

Upto 90g per hour for events > 3hrs

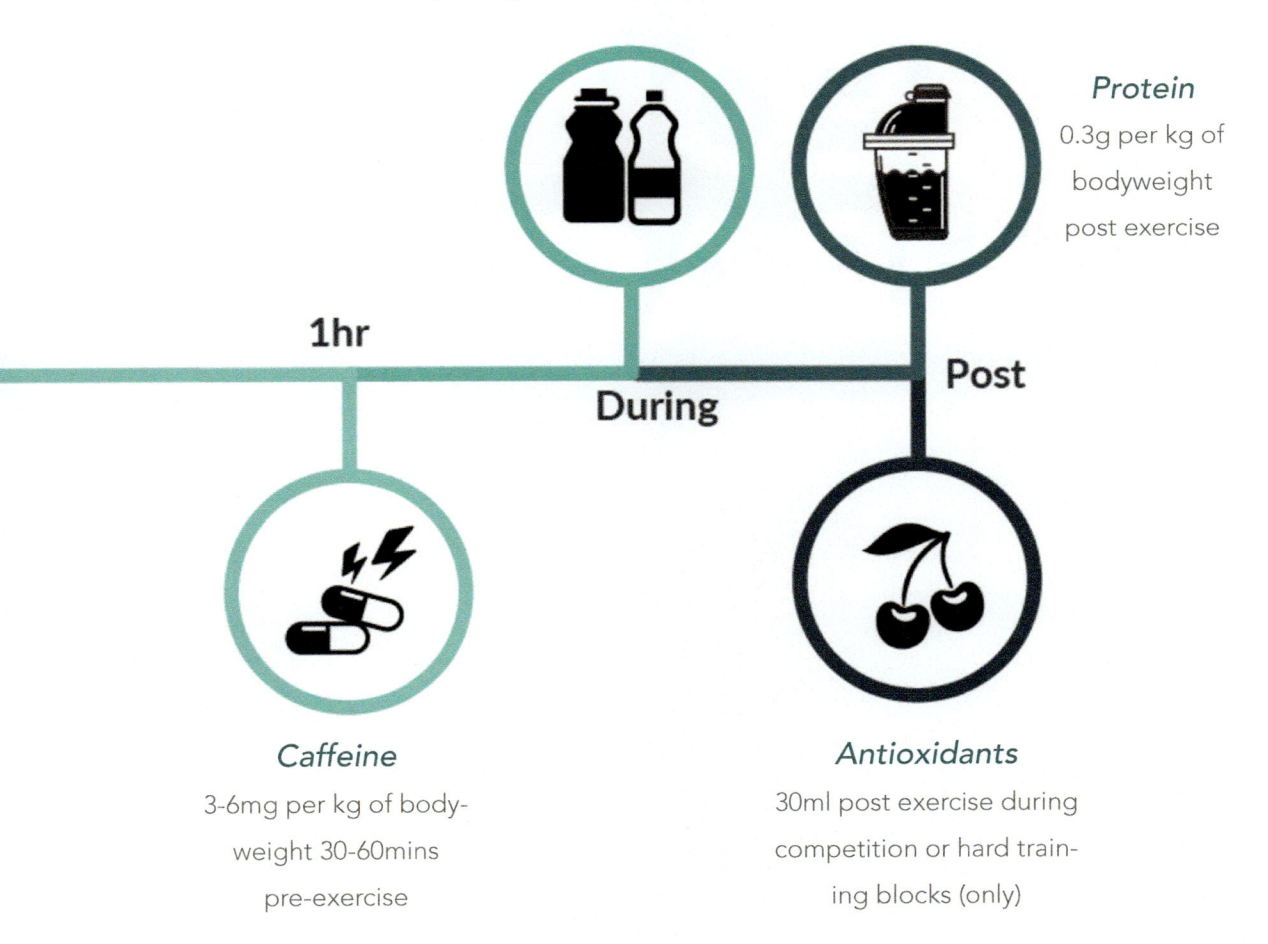

Protein

0.3g per kg of bodyweight post exercise

1hr — **During** — **Post**

Caffeine

3-6mg per kg of bodyweight 30-60mins pre-exercise

Antioxidants

30ml post exercise during competition or hard training blocks (only)

Supplements

CHAPTER FIVE
THEORY TO PRACTICE

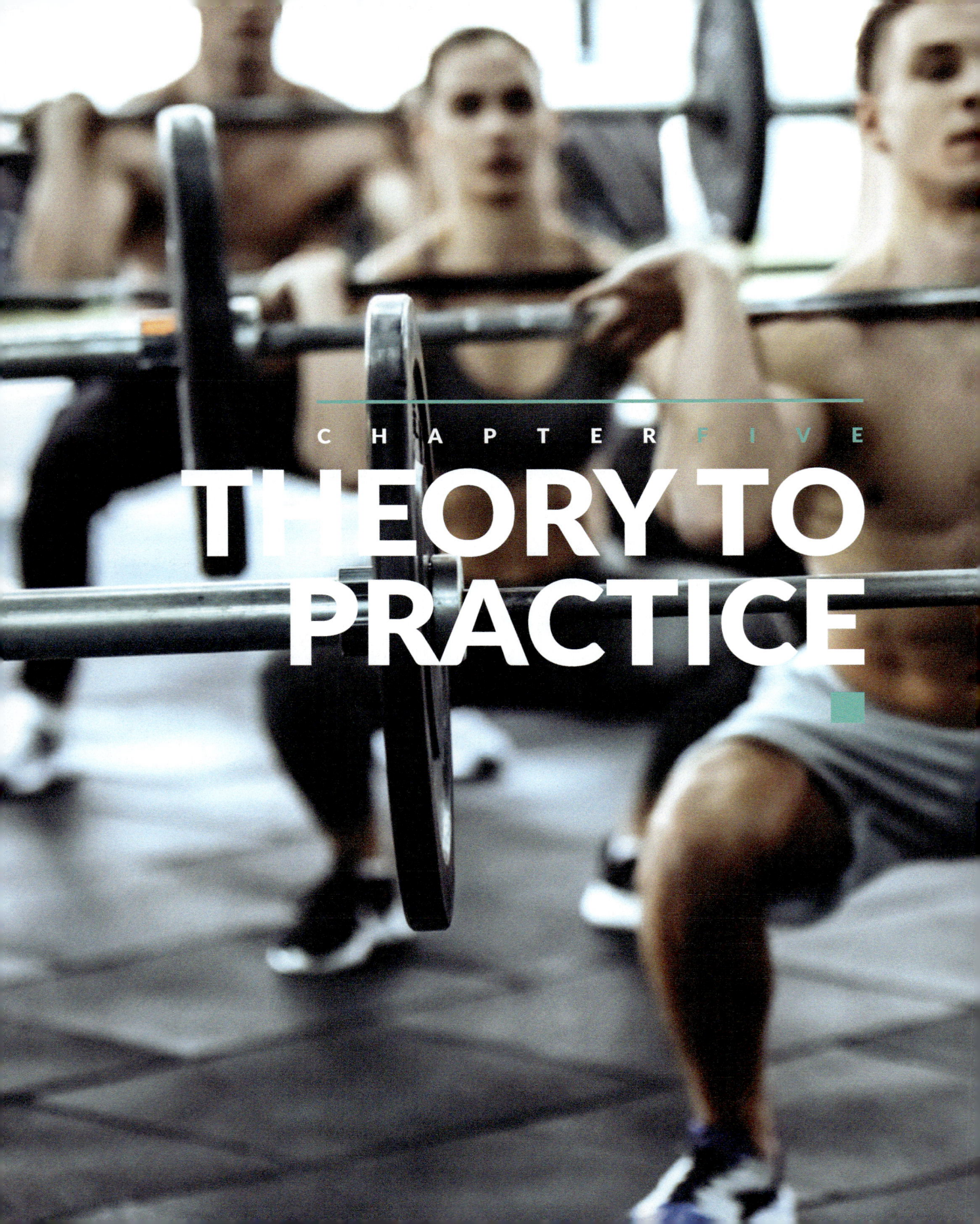

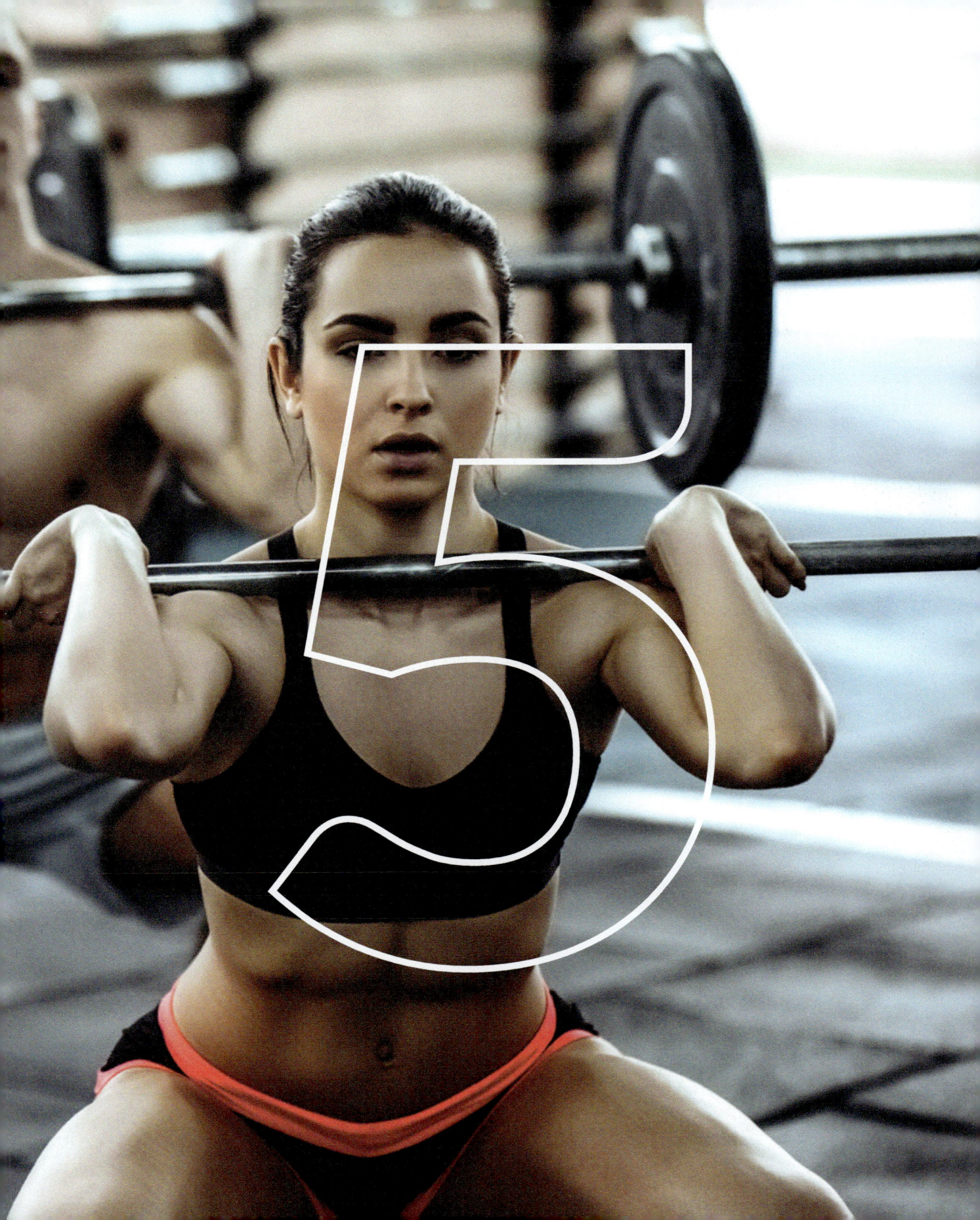

5

5.1 PLANNING YOUR DIET

Before we start it is important to consider what your current situation is and what your goals are. Whether your current goal is performance, weight loss or weight gain, the long-term objective should be to implement a healthy dietary practice that you can stick to forever. Therefore, it's important to understand your goals and set realistic expectations.

Planning your diet

If you're looking to shed a couple of pounds, then a little attention to tidying up your diet should be enough to bring about noticeable change. However, if you want to reach a higher level of competitiveness and affect your performance in a meaningful way, you will have to make some more impactful changes.

In case you do not have a specific goal in mind, we recommend that you plan to have an endpoint or a date to work towards. This could be a competition, a holiday or even a photoshoot. Having a goal like this gives you something to keep focus on and work towards. We recommend a period of 12 weeks to notice changes in dietary habits, body composition and performance. This will, of course, vary from person to person but this time frame gives you room to cement good dietary practice.

DIETARY EXPECTATIONS

Fat loss

Although rapid weight loss can be a strong motivation, a large kcal deficit can lead to a more significant reduction in muscle mass and performance compared to slower rates of weight loss (1). The likelihood of sticking to an extreme diet is also very small and such severe measures can lead to physical and psychological problems such as low self-esteem, poor body image, illness and injury. Being able to stick to an eating pattern for the foreseeable future is key for long-term success. Therefore, you should focus on a smaller and more manageable drop in kcals, which will make dieting feel a lot less like dieting. This will help you stay with your plan for longer.

How quickly should you expect results?

Your rate of weight loss will depend on your current body fat percentage and exercise activity. A higher body fat percentage will result in a quicker loss of weight whereas a lower initial body fat percentage will result in slower weight loss. As a guide, you should hope to expect a loss of between 0.5-1% of your bodyweight per week. If retaining a level of performance is also a priority, then a slower rate of weight loss will be more desirable (2).

Example - 90kg athlete

A target rate of weight loss will be between 0.45-0.9kg per week, based on 0.5-1% of bodyweight per week.

0.5% of bodyweight = (90/100 x 0.5) = 0.45kg per week.
1% of bodyweight = (90/100 x 1) = 0.9kg per week.

Diet length

Trying to lose weight as an athlete can be an issue when you also want to maintain certain levels of performance. When reducing kcals and creating an energy deficit, the body does what it can to preserve the status quo, whereby through something called adaptive thermogenesis (AT), it reduces energy expenditure to prevent further weight loss. This not only inhibits fat loss but can also be detrimental to performance.

Basically – your body doesn't make it easy to lose weight

Why does this happen?
- *A drop in lean mass results in a reduction in Resting Energy Expenditure (REE). You don't burn as many kcals at rest*
- *Hormonal responses (leptin, insulin, testosterone, ghrelin) to a hypocaloric diet (lower kcals than you need) also promotes hunger, reduces metabolic rate, which makes it difficult to maintain muscle*
- *A reduction in muscle mass requires less energy to perform activity reducing the number of kcals being used. For example, a man weighing 90kg will require more energy to run compared to a 50kg woman*
- *NEAT, or the kcals expended through none exercise activities (fidgeting and moving around) also decreases*

To help counter this, you must look to reduce these responses by making further small incremental changes to your diet when progress stalls, utilising small kcal deficits and following a strict strength programme.

However, you can't be expected to do this forever. This is why you may want to adopt a phased approach to your dieting.

What is a phased approach?

Dieting for lengthy periods can lead to muscle loss, a performance decrement, poor sleep, increased hunger and fatigue. For this reason, we recommend staying in an energy deficit for no more than 12-16 weeks.

A phased approach is a method of breaking your diet into periods of eating in a kcal deficit (dieting phase) and eating in a kcal surplus (muscle gain and maintenance phase).

A maintenance phase is a practical way to give you a psychological but also a physical break from dieting. These maintenance phases of increased kcals enable hormones to reset to normal levels that can reduce hunger, cravings, increase energy levels, metabolic rate and improve training. This can result in more favourable long-term changes in body composition and performance. From a psychological perspective, it also gives you a break from tracking and simply dieting. It's not always fun eating in a kcal deficit!

After 12-16 weeks of dieting, we recommend you then follow a maintenance phase that lasts around 6-12 weeks. The longer you diet for, the longer your maintenance phase should be. This will give your body plenty of time to recover before you choose to diet again.

Example Fat loss plan

January	February	March	April	May	June	July
Fat loss	Fat loss	Fat loss	Maintenance	Fat loss	Fat loss	Maintenance

Theory To Practice

Weight gain expectations

Unlike fat loss, muscle gain can take longer to achieve. Favourable body composition should be important for the athletes which is why only a moderate kcal surplus is recommended. If building muscle is your priority, then following a strict training programme is also key.

Training status	Potential gains
Beginner	1-1.5% of bodyweight per month (able to progress their lifts on a weekly basis)
Intermediate	0.5-1% of bodyweight per month (able to progress their lifts on a monthly basis)
Advanced	Less than 0.5% of bodyweight per month (able to progress their lifts over a few months)

(3. Taken from Eric Helms and the Muscle and Strength Pyramids 2017).

Similar to weight loss, you should still only look to stay in a weight gain phase for a set length of time. Being in a kcal surplus for extended periods can lead to increased body fat %, fat cell hyperplasia (multiplication of fat cells), a decrement in performance and health. For these reasons, we recommend your weight gain phases should only last between 8-18 weeks. This gives you enough time to build muscle without exacerbating any of the negative side effects listed above. We also recommend that you don't enter a dieting phase immediately after finishing a period of building muscle, but instead transition into a maintenance phase for at least 2 weeks to help prevent any muscle loss.

January	February	March	April	May
Muscle gain	Muscle gain	Muscle gain	Muscle gain	Maintenance

In chapter 12 (Adjusting Your Diet) we go through the steps of how to make the transition effectively from either a fat loss or building phase to a maintenance phase.

Can you build muscle and lose fat simultaneously?

Even though it's possible to increase lean mass in a kcal deficit (4), it's more beneficial to focus on a kcal surplus to facilitate greater change in muscle mass and to support your training demands (5). If fat loss is more of a priority, then start with a small kcal deficit. Other compensations must be made by increasing strength training and protein intake to support muscle retention.

This is the reason why we recommend starting your plan at a maintenance set of kcals. This enables you to diet on the maximum number of kcals possible where depending on your results from these 4 weeks, you can then make a choice to either enter a fat loss or muscle gain phase.

Jan	Feb	Mar	Apr	May	Jun	Jul	Aug	Sep	Oct	Nov	Dec
Maintain	Fat loss				Maintain		Muscle gain				Maintain

Performance - How to plan your training year?

When planning your training year, you must first consider your primary goal.
- *Are you looking to lose weight?*
- *Are you looking to improve body composition?*
- *Are you looking to increase strength?*
- *Are you looking to work on your endurance?*
- *Are you looking to compete at a particular event?*

At Box, we like to use a radar chart like the one below to help build a better idea of which areas the athlete needs most attention.

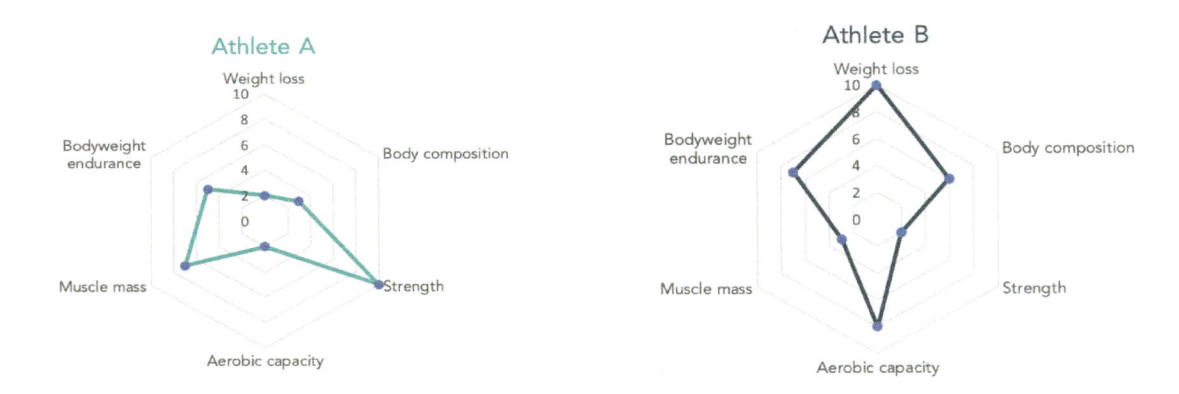

Based on this analysis, you can decide the area you wish to focus on, or how you will periodise your nutrition alongside your training plan. From the chart on the previous page, we can see that athlete A needs to focus on weight loss, body composition and endurance. Athlete B needs to work on strength and increasing muscle mass.

Example yearly training plan - Athlete A

Athlete A wants to perform at his best for 'The Open' in February. His other priority is to lose weight and improve body composition. Based on this, we can adapt his nutrition throughout the year to ensure improvements in his body composition without compromising performance for The Open.

Jan	Feb	Mar	Apr	May	Jun	Jul	Aug	Sep	Oct	Nov	Dec
Phase 5			Off	Phase 1			Phase 2	Phase 3		Phase 4	
Perform			Off	Fat loss			Main-te-nance	Strength		Endurance	

Phase 1 – Fat loss
Nutrition considerations
- Eat to lose weight - Eat in a kcal deficit
- Keep protein to the higher end of the spectrum
- Include some fasted endurance sessions for adaptation. See chapter 2 for more on 'Training low'

Phase 2 – Maintenance
Nutrition considerations
- Bring kcals ups to a maintenance level to match the work being performed

Phase 3 – Strength
Nutrition considerations
- Eat to gain weight. Eat in a small kcal surplus
- Prioritise protein and carbohydrates around sessions for fuel and recovery
- Supplement with creatine

Phase 4 – Endurance
Nutrition considerations
- Focus on carbohydrates around high intensity sessions
- Use a low carb approach for long easier endurance-based work
- Keep protein high to help maintain muscle mass

Phase 5 – Perform
Nutrition considerations
- Eat to perform. Eat at a maintenance level and match kcals to the work being performed
- Focus on recovery and fuelling sessions correctly

Example yearly training plan - Athlete B

Athlete B has entered a number of competitions and is looking to compete throughout the summer. Her major weakness is her strength, so the majority of her training year will be spent improving this area.

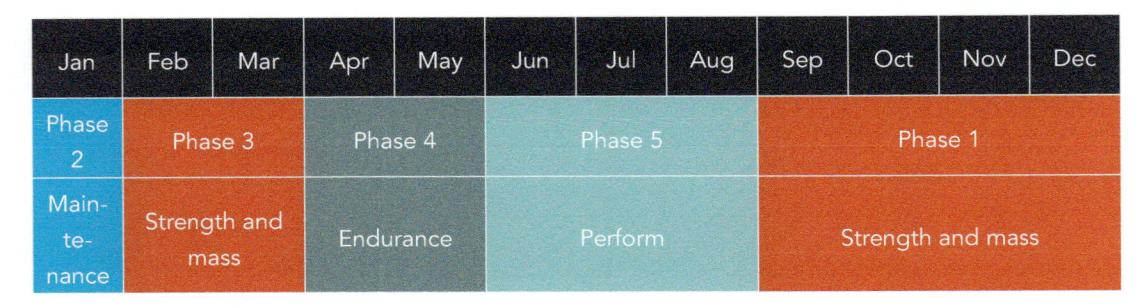

Jan	Feb	Mar	Apr	May	Jun	Jul	Aug	Sep	Oct	Nov	Dec
Phase 2	Phase 3		Phase 4		Phase 5			Phase 1			
Maintenance	Strength and mass		Endurance		Perform			Strength and mass			

Phase 1 – Strength and mass
Nutrition considerations
- Eat to grow. Eat in a large kcal surplus
- Prioritise protein and carbohydrates around sessions for fuel and recovery
- Supplement with creatine

Phase 2 – Maintenance
Nutrition considerations
- Bring kcals down to a maintenance level to match the work being performed

Phase 3 – Strength
Nutrition considerations
- Bring kcals back up to a small kcal surplus
- Prioritise protein and carbohydrates around sessions for fuel and recovery

Phase 4 – Endurance
Nutrition considerations
- Focus on carbohydrates around sessions for fuel and recovery
- Keep protein high to help maintain muscle mass

Phase 5 – Perform

Nutrition considerations

- Eat at a maintenance level and match kcals to the work being performed
- Focus on recovery and fuelling sessions correctly

Example yearly training plan - Athlete C

Athlete C has no particular goal. He is a well-rounded athlete and wants to be able to compete whenever he chooses. He follows a mixed modal programme where he looks to develop all areas of his fitness simultaneously.

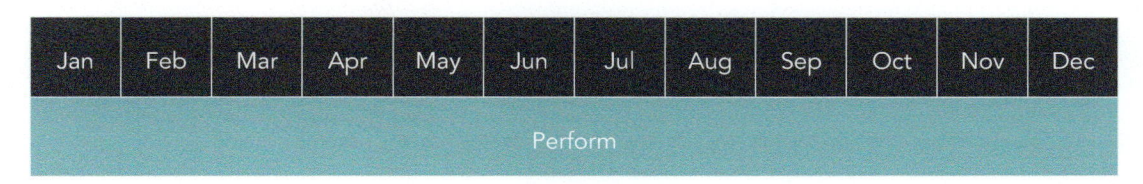

Jan	Feb	Mar	Apr	May	Jun	Jul	Aug	Sep	Oct	Nov	Dec
Perform											

Nutrition considerations

- Match kcals with the work required
- Follow a weekly periodised approach by fuelling each session based on its caloric needs. Look back at chapter 2 (daily carbohydrate needs) for help with adjusting your fuelling based on your training

Example periodised approach to fuelling training sessions

Activity	Fuelling strategy
Rest	Low fuel low carb
Low volume (less than 6 reps) resistance training. Powerlifting/ Olympic weightlifting. Gymnastic sessions.	Moderate fuel low carb
Aerobic capacity work/endurance training	Moderate fuel moderate carb
Metabolic conditioning/High intensity interval training/ High volume resistance or circuit training	Moderate fuel moderate carb
Training twice in one day	High fuel high carb

Example weekly periodistaion

Day	Activity	Fuelling strategy
Monday	Weightlifting	Moderate fuel low carb
Tuesday	WOD	Moderate fuel moderate carb
Wednesday	WOD (am) Weightlifting (pm)	High fuel high carb
Thursday	Rest	Low fuel low carb
Friday	WOD	Moderate fuel moderate carb
Saturday	WOD	Moderate fuel moderate carb
Sunday	Rest	Low fuel low carb

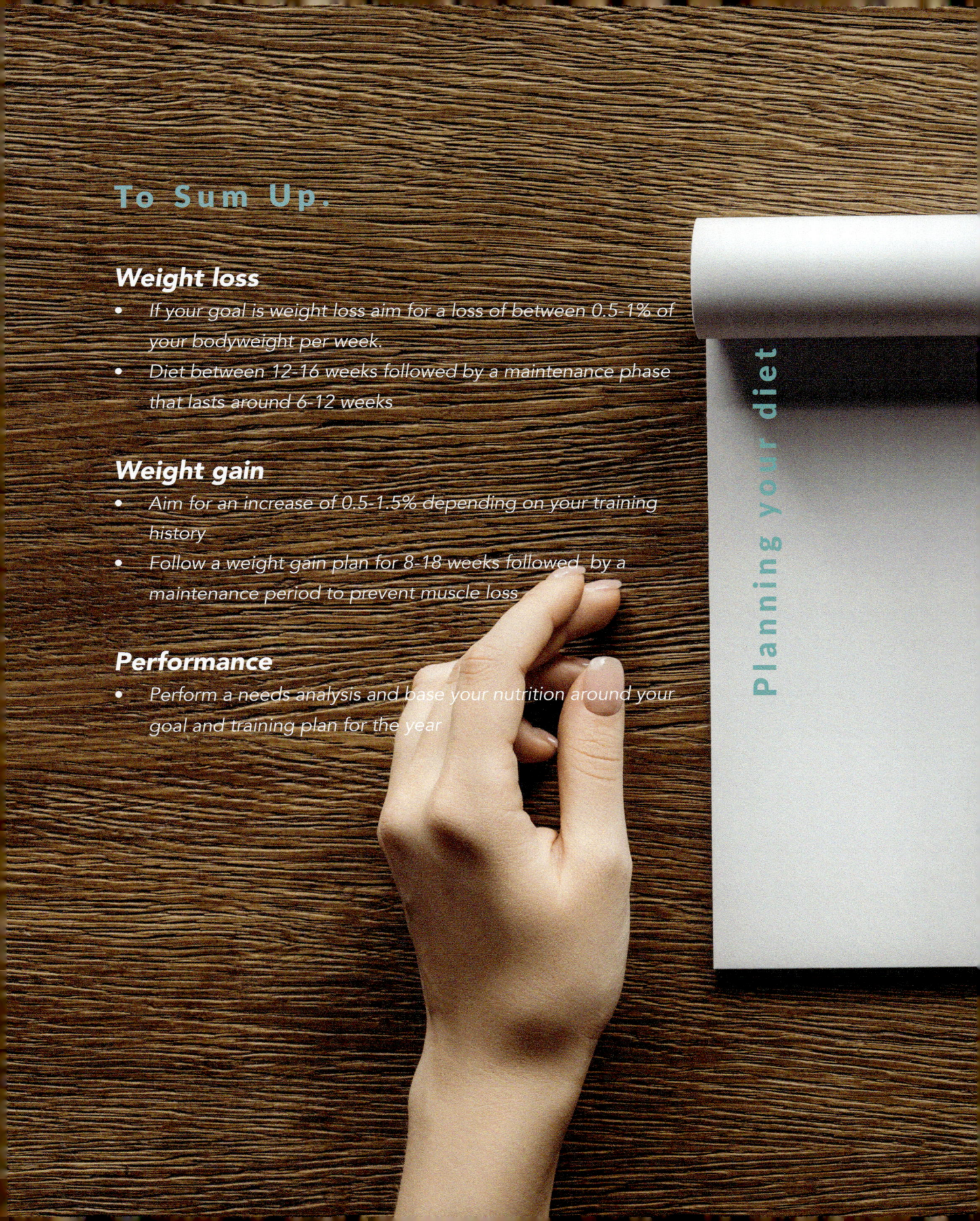

To Sum Up.

Weight loss
- *If your goal is weight loss aim for a loss of between 0.5-1% of your bodyweight per week.*
- *Diet between 12-16 weeks followed by a maintenance phase that lasts around 6-12 weeks*

Weight gain
- *Aim for an increase of 0.5-1.5% depending on your training history*
- *Follow a weight gain plan for 8-18 weeks followed by a maintenance period to prevent muscle loss*

Performance
- *Perform a needs analysis and base your nutrition around your goal and training plan for the year*

Planning your diet

CHAPTER SIX

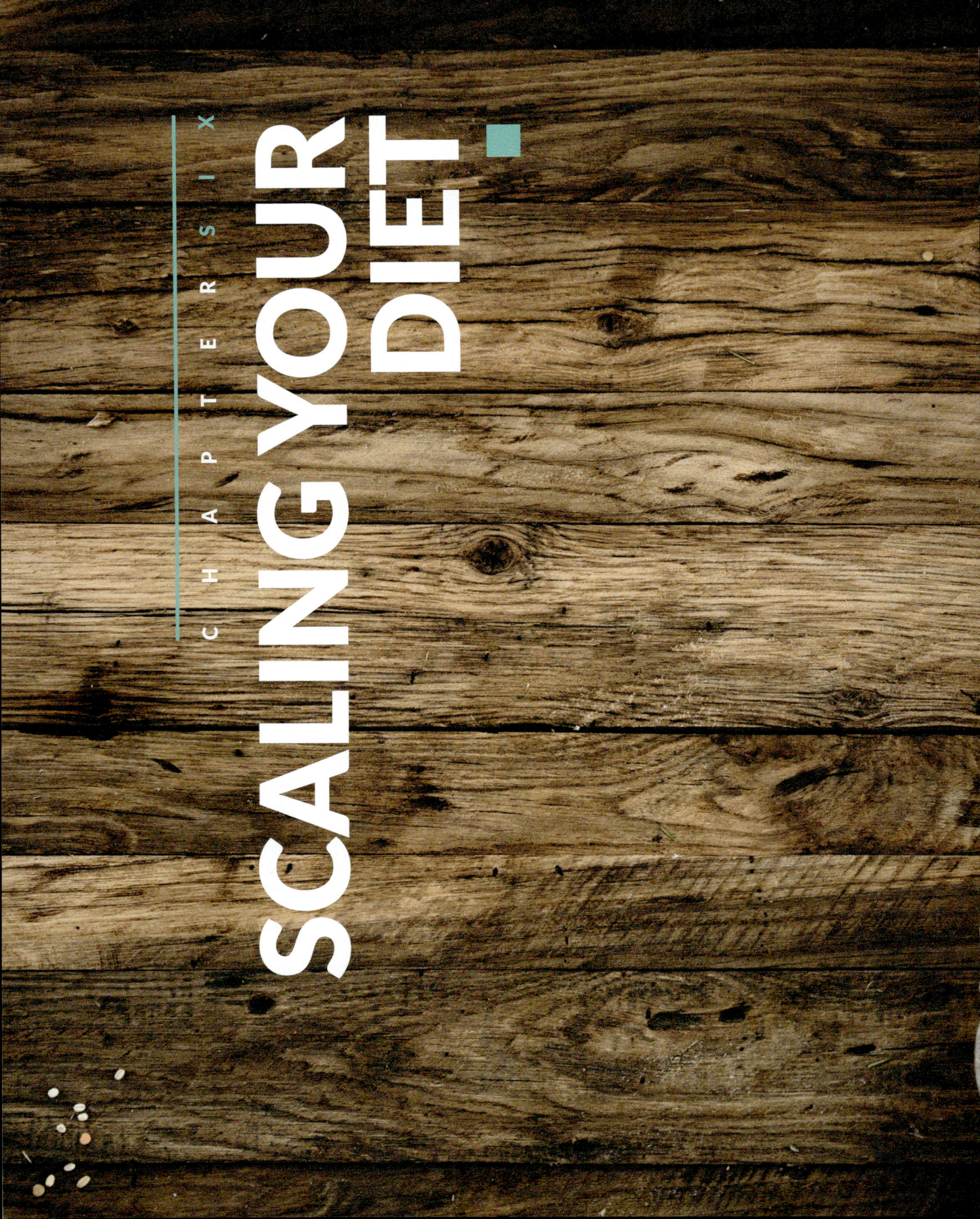

SCALING YOUR DIET

6

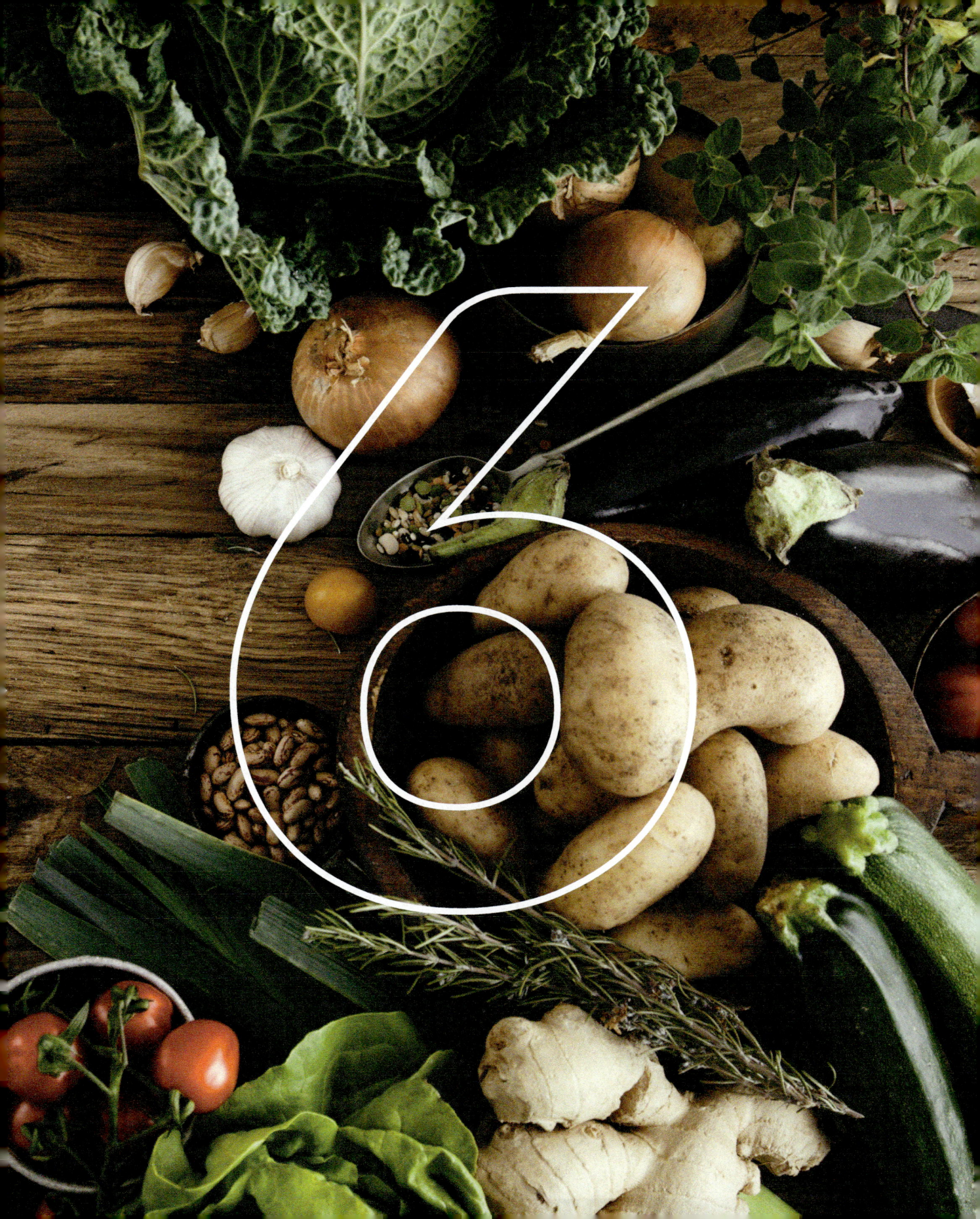

At Box we follow a framework that enables you to scale up your diet whether you're completely new to nutrition or you're an athlete who is looking to compete at the highest level. Whatever your starting point, the idea is to systematically find ways to improve your diet wherever you can.

Level 1 - The habit-based approach

One of the fundamentals of the Box framework is to understand the Box Basics, which are a selection of habits we will be going through later on in the chapter. These practices help build the foundations of a better diet, whether the goal is performance, to look better, or just feel better.

If you struggle with the idea of tracking your food, or still find it difficult to grasp the "ins and outs" of what good nutrition is, these simple habits enable you to focus on one or two things at any one given time. As you begin to embrace these habits, your diet will begin to take shape.

Level 2 - Scaling up your diet - Using your numbers

We encourage people to know their numbers, or how many kcals and macronutrients they require for their training goals.

Although you don't have to track kcals and macronutrients to see results, it's an incredibly powerful tool to help you understand the values of food and how to adjust your eating based on your progress.

This is also a time when you will want to start practising with fuelling and recovery strategies for your training.

Level 3 - Complete intuition

After tracking your food and performance for a few weeks, you will begin to get a better grasp of how much you are eating and how much you should be eating. You will also begin to figure out your own personal nutrition strategies based on training and competition goals.

Once you believe you are beginning to see change by following this approach, it is time to start moving away from tracking and become more intuitive with what you eat. Learning to listen to body cues like hunger and tiredness rather than emotion or responses to a situation is a useful skill to develop. In addition, recording how you feel when you train will also enable you to eat in accordance with what your body needs, rather than blindly following a set number or figures, or swaying to emotions.

This is also a time when you should consider more advanced strategies such as 'training low' (Chapter 2) or adding supplementation to your diet.

6.1 THE HABIT BASED APPROACH

Although awareness of nutritional values (kcals, protein, carbs, fats) is fundamental for progress, habits are key to sustained change. This is the reason why as part of the Box framework, we look at developing several habits that help form the basis of a good diet. As you begin to implement these habits, your healthy diet begins to take shape and results will follow.

Habit checklist - Athlete fundamentals

1. Include more vegetables
You may see this as a recurring theme but a diet rich in a variety of vegetables has numerous benefits for health, body composition and performance. So make consuming a variety of different coloured vegetables in your diet a priority.

2. Drink more water
Hydrate yourself. An incredibly simple way to boost performance, help control cravings, improve energy levels and mood. Aim to drink water immediately upon waking and until your urine becomes transparent. Or just make sure you always keep a water bottle with you.

3. Make hitting protein numbers a priority

The literature consistently shows us that a diet high in protein helps with favourable changes in body composition and building new muscle. If you prefer not to calculate this number, aim to consume a portion (20-30g for women, 30-40g for men) of protein with every meal.

4. Educate yourself to help make better food choices and substitution

Investing some time into understanding the foods that you're eating will enable you to make better food choices and help you identify areas where you need to improve. By understanding the nutritional values of food like the number of kcals, protein or fat they contain will give you a better grasp of how much you are currently eating, and also how much you should be eating. This gives you more flexibility with your diet moving forward.

The best way to do this is simply to track what you eat.

5. Start by adding foods in rather than only taking foods out

Increasing foods like sources of lean protein, fibrous fruit and vegetables will have just as much of an impact on performance and body composition as removing all typically 'bad' foods such as biscuits, cakes, ice cream and chocolate. It will also help with reducing the feeling of 'dieting' and increasing the feeling of fullness. This will help you stick to your new eating plan.

6. Get 7-8hrs of sleep

Sleep is just as important as nutrition and exercise. The foundation for recovery, sleep helps with the revitalisation of both physical and mental function. Being deprived of sleep can have a negative impact on body composition, hunger, hormone regulation, cognitive function, energy levels, risk of illness and injury and also lead to a drop in performance. If you can't get 7-8 hours of sleep daily, consider power naps (aim for 15-20 minutes) when you can.

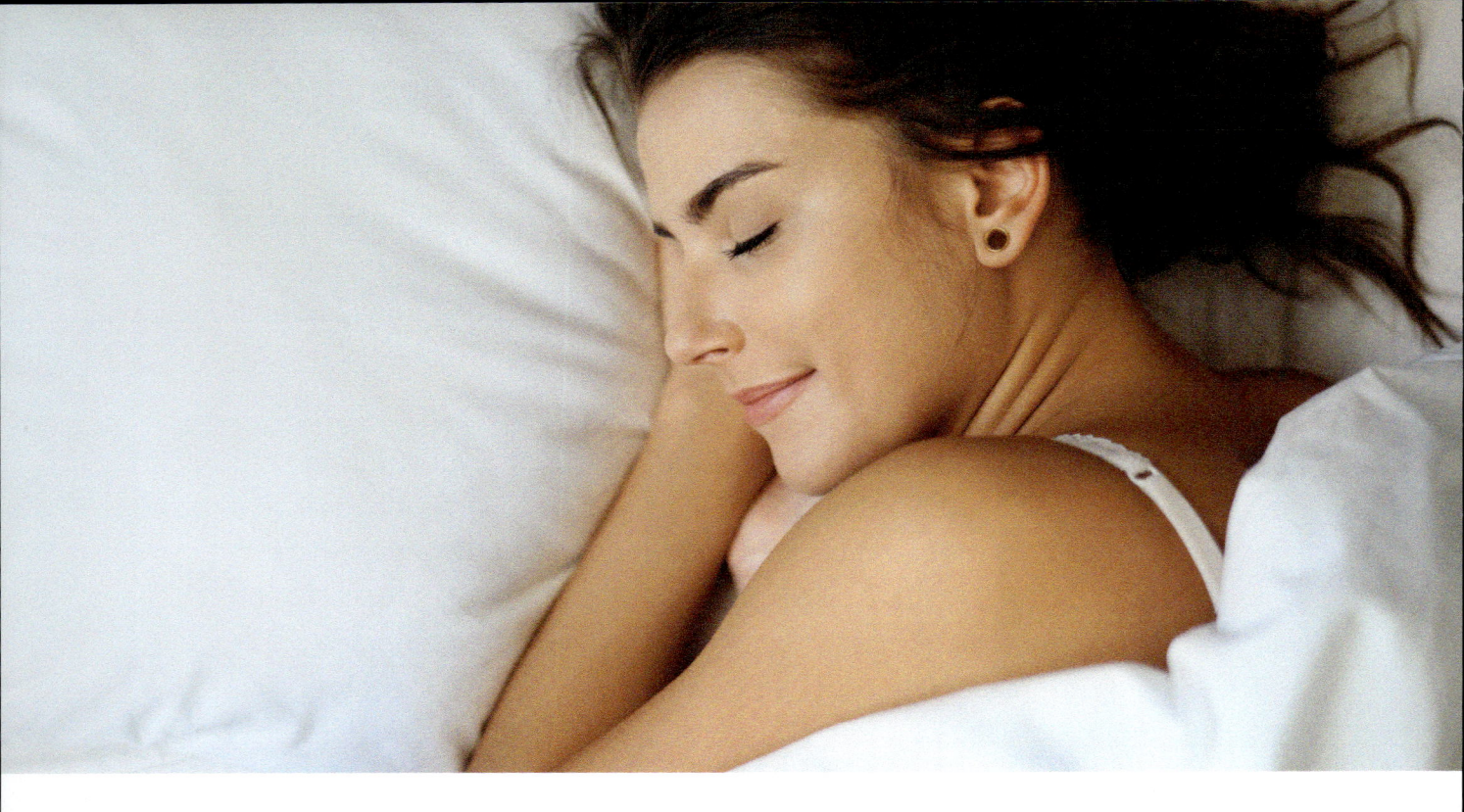

Tips for a good night's sleep

1. Spend more time outside

Daily sunlight can improve sleep quality (6) so make time to go for a walk or even exercise outdoors.

2. Reduce coffee and other stimulants later in the day

Caffeine can be present in the body up to 8hrs after consumption, which for some can negatively affect the quality of sleep (7).

3. Have a proper sleep schedule

Make the effort to go to bed and wake up at the same time each day. Having a set sleeping schedule can help with long term sleep quality (8), whereas irregular sleep patterns can alter the circadian rhythm. This is the process that helps align the body with sunrise and sunset.

4. Avoid alcohol
Alcohol can disrupt sleep quality and sleep patterns (9) so try and limit daily alcohol consumption.

5. Take a bath
A warm bath or shower before bed is an effective way to relax the body and improve sleep quality (10).

6. Invest
The quality of your mattress and pillows can have a positive impact on sleep quality, especially for those who suffer with back and neck pain (11, 12).

7. Make your room comfortable
A relaxing space to sleep that is cool, free from noise and bright lights can have a positive effect on sleep quality (13).

8. Reduce blue light
Light emitted from laptops, smart phones and tablets in the evening can prevent you from relaxing and reaching deep sleep (14). Download the app F.Lux to remove the blue light on your laptop. There are similar apps available for your smart phone.

9. Relax
Strategies such as reading a book, meditation/mindfulness, massage or listening to music can help relax the body and mind leading to better quality of sleep (15).

10. Don't exercise late
Although exercise can have a positive effect on sleep, working out just before you go to bed may delay sleeping as a result of alertness and hormones such as adrenaline and epinephrine being released (16).

Weight loss checklist

1. Reduce added sugar
Although sugar is not inherently bad, too much is. Added sugar increases palatability of foods that reduce satiation and increases the likelihood of over- eating. Make a conscious effort to consume less than 10 percent of kcals per day from added sugars, unless training volume is high (endurance-based activities that last longer than 90 mins or training twice per day).

2. Try not to drink your kcals
Liquid kcals quickly add up and often go under the radar. This means you often won't be aware of how many kcals you have consumed in this way. Have you ever checked how many kcals are in your vanilla latte or your 'healthy' fruit smoothie? It's worth knowing! Choose water, low fat milk and low kcal options where possible.

3. Reduce high sugar/high fat condiments
As with drinking your kcals, the consumption of too many condiments like ketchup, mayonnaise and salad dressings can have a negative influence on body composition and potentially performance goals. That's not to say you can't have them, just be aware of how much you're consuming.

4. Watch your portion sizes
Use the weight loss plate and main meal portion recommendations to form the basis of your meals (Chapter 9).

5. Practise mindful eating
Remove distractions such as the TV and scrolling through your phone whilst eating, as this type of behaviour can lead to consuming more. Instead, listen to your body and stop when you're almost full, chew your food, eat slowly and enjoy it.

6. Consider NEAT
None Exercise Activity Thermogenesis (NEAT - subconscious movement kcal expenditure) and None Exercise Physical Activity levels (NEPA - intentional movement that doesn't include formal exercise) can play a large part in whether you lose or gain weight. In fact, these can make up to 2000 kcals difference between people of a similar size (17). Therefore, although not terribly accurate, the use of a fitness wearable can be beneficial when trying to calculate your energy expenditure for the day. Or, you can 'guestimate' by multiplying your BMR by an activity factor. We recommend you aim for 10,000 steps per day and potentially more if you are struggling to lose weight.

Simple swaps for weight loss
- Black coffee instead of a latte
- Lemon juice and balsamic dressing instead of mayonnaise or salad cream
- Water instead of fizzy drinks
- Greek yoghurt instead of ice cream
- ½ your nut butter portion

Weight gain checklist

1. Prioritise recovery
Ensure that you consume a carbohydrate and protein rich snack immediately after you train. Also include a protein rich snack before bed (smoothie, cheese on crackers, oats with milk).

2. Eat regularly
Optimise muscle protein synthesis (building and recovery) and help kcal intake by eating every 2-3 hours.

3. Carbohydrate choices

Sugary foods such as honey, jam, malt loaf and flapjacks prior to training are good ways to increase your carbohydrate intake and help with performance. Likewise, consuming these types of foods after you train helps with glycogen synthesis and recovery. Also strive to substitute your carbohydrate choices for higher kcal ones, for instance pasta instead of rice, bagels instead of bread and granola instead of oats.

4. Add more healthy fats

Fat is an easy way to consume more kcals. Use olive oil more often when cooking, add butter to vegetables, choose fattier cuts of meat and dairy. Also try to include nut butters as part of your snacks.

5. Utilise liquid nutrition

Smoothies, recovery shakes and intra-workout drinks are an easy way to increase kcals without the feeling of being overly full.

6. Consider Supplements

If you cannot meet your kcal and macronutrient targets with food alone, consider using creatine, a weight gain supplement and protein powder.

Making these habits stick

To help implement some of these practices, we have included a habit tracker (right) in the resource section (https://boxnutrition.co.uk/fuellingresources) to note down habits you need to work on. These could include eating vegetables with all your main meals, drinking 8 glasses of water every day or reducing alcohol to two evenings per week. Make them pertinent to you and your goals.

Examples:

Habit	Date	1	2	3	4	5	6	7	Notes
Increase water intake to 2-4L	01/01	Y	Y	Y	N	Y	N	N	Make sure I take a water bottle to work with me
Record your weight and measurements	08/01	Y	Y	Y	Y	Y	Y	N	
Track what you eat every day									
Have fruit or veg with every meal and snack									
Remover sugary drinks									
Remove sugar from tea and coffee									
Stay within your calories									
Hit your protein targets for the day									
Hit your carbohydrates targets for the day									
Hit your fat targets for the day									
Reduce unhealthy foods to 'X' times per week									
Reduce eating out to 'X' times per week									
Get 7-8 hrs of sleep/get to bed by 22:00									
Hit 'X' steps per day									
Reduce condiments									

Scaling Your Diet

In search of marginal gains

Over the last decade the term marginal gains has been popularised by Sir David Brailsford, the UK and what was Team Sky's cycling director, who was accredited for the surge in British cycling success.

His marginal gains philosophy was to look at all aspects of cycling that could be attributed to better performance and identify ways of making small improvements. The idea is that just a 1% adjustment in numerous areas will lead to a larger overall gain. These could include advancements in bikes, clothing, nutrition, psychology and recovery.

Results don't lie. The UK has become one of, if not the powerhouse of world track cycling and Team Sky recorded six out of the last seven Tour De' France victories. A remarkable feat considering the obscurity of British cycling in previous years.

This idea of marginal gains can be applied to any area performance. Similar to the habit-based approach we use at Box, identify factors that may contribute to success and systematically look for ways to make adjustments where you can. This could be getting a better mattress to help with sleep, a water bottle with a fruit infuser to help you drink more, a set of measuring cups to help gauge your portion sizes or a planner to help with your preparation. These are a just a few of many examples that could help you with your own marginal gains.

Improvement

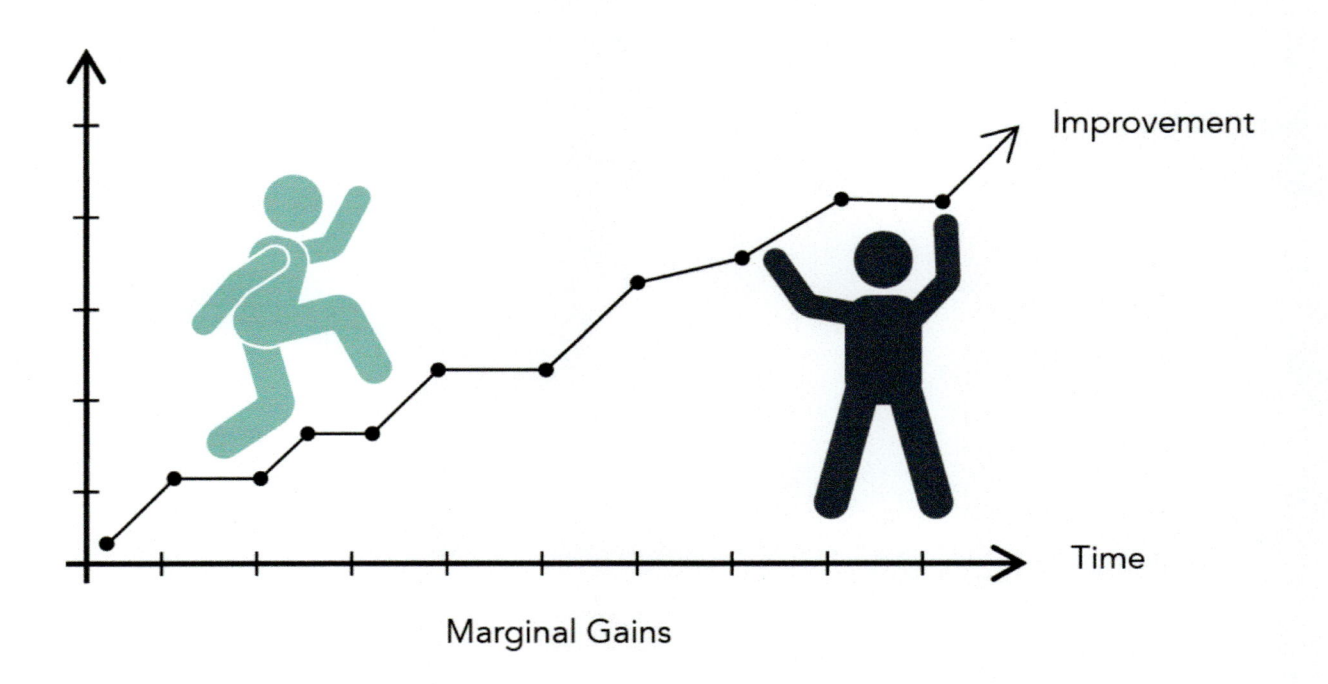

Time

Marginal Gains

Scaling Your Diet

7

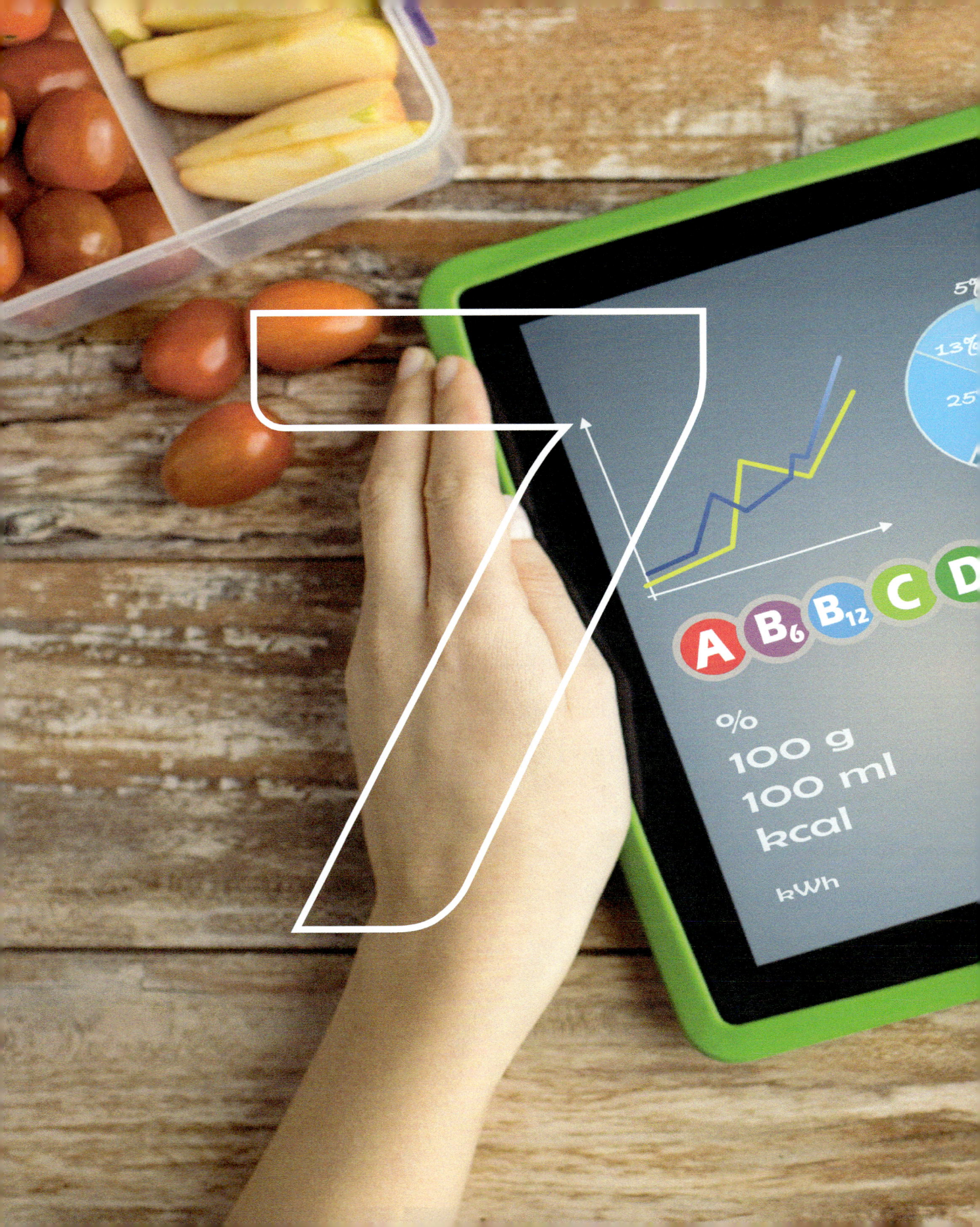

CHAPTER SEVEN

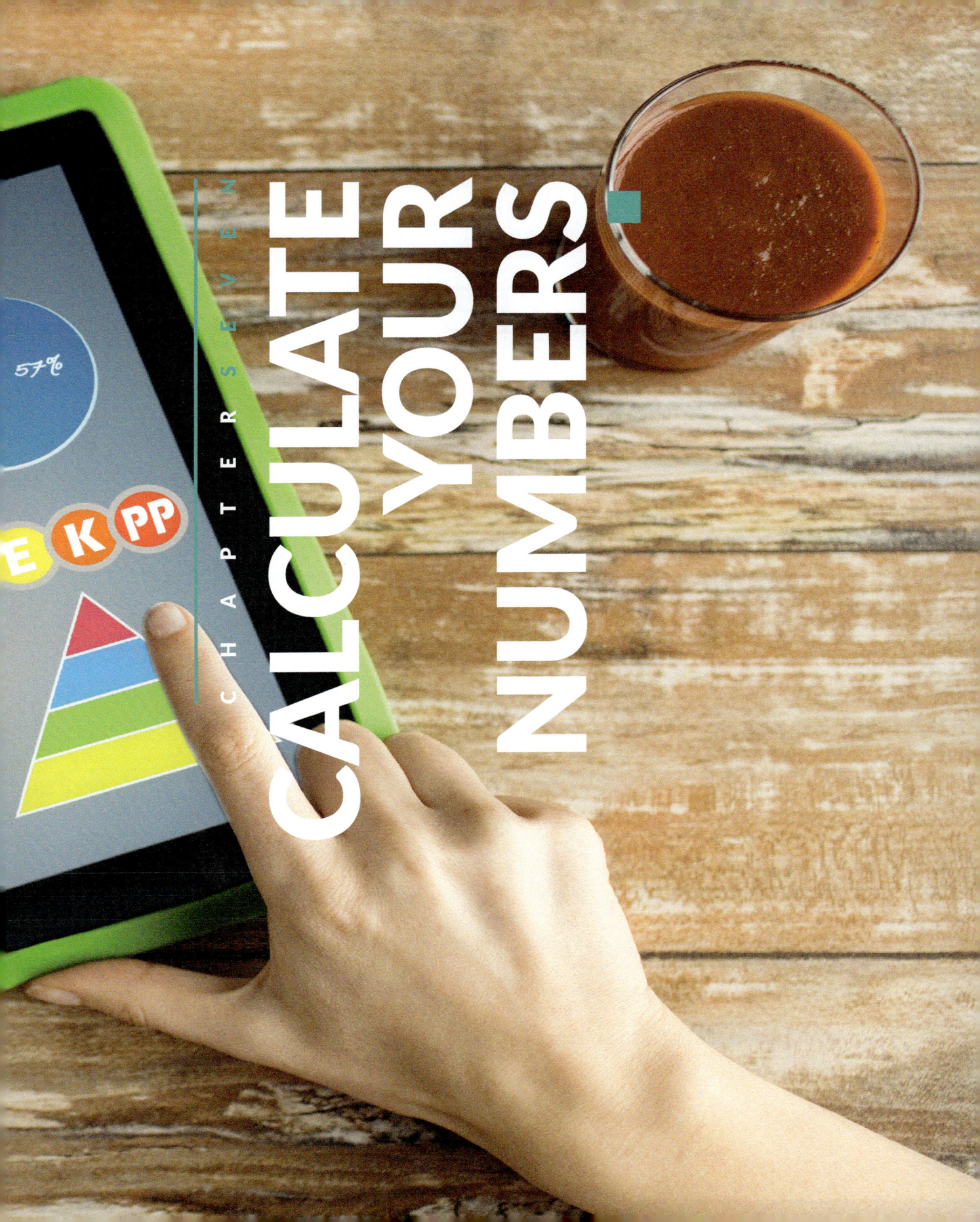

CALCULATE YOUR NUMBERS

7.1 CALCULATE YOUR NUMBERS

Once you have begun to lay the foundations of your diet using some of the habits listed in the previous chapter, you should then consider taking things a step further by calculating your kcal and macronutrient targets.

The first section of this book went through the theory behind how to calculate your nutritional values. This section will teach you how to work out your target sets of numbers step-by-step.

Calculate your kcal needs

Step 1 - Calculate your BMR

The first step is working out your BMR by using the Katch-Mcardle formula:

BMR = 370 + (21.6 x Lean Body Mass(kg))
Lean Body Mass = (Weight(kg) x (100-(Body Fat %)))/100

To help calculate your body fat percentage use the US Navy calculator:

https://www.calculator.net/body-fat-calculator.html

We go in to further details about your body fat percentage in Chapter 12 (Measuring Your Progress).

Step 2 - Calculate your daily energy expenditure

Calculate your daily energy expenditure by estimating your Physical Activity Level (PAL). This is a rough measure of your lifestyle activity and does not include planned or structured exercise but only day-to-day life. Unless you have an active job, set your PAL at sedentary (we will later calculate activity from exercise).

PAL
- Mostly inactive or sedentary: 1.2
- Fairly active: 1.3
- Moderately active: 1.4
- Active: 1.5
- Very active: 1.7

Step 3 - Estimate energy expenditure through exercise

Estimate the number of kcals you will expend during exercise using the MET scale or with the use a fitness wearable.

Each day of the week can be defined by the amount of activity performed. A recovery day or day without a workout would be classed as a "light day". Training once would be classified as a "moderate day", and days where you train twice would be classed as "hard days".

What about the Thermic Effect of Feeding (TEF)?

Although TEF can account for an additional 5-10% of your Total Energy Expenditure (TEE), this is only a rough estimate, as the amount and type of food you eat will alter this number. Protein has a far higher TEF than carbohydrates and fat. Roughly 25% of the kcals from protein eaten will be lost as heat, whereas only around 70–75% will be absorbed. Carbohydrates may lose 10% as heat, whereas fat may only lose 2-3%. As this figure will vary day-to-day and only has a small bearing on your TEE, we therefore recommend not to worry too much about the impact of TEF.

If you struggle to put on weight or you want to be as accurate as possible with your starting estimates, then you may want to account for TEF by adding 5-10% to your TEE.

Step 4: Adjust for body composition goals

Add the figures from steps 2 and 3. This is the number of kcals you need to maintain your body weight.

- *If your goal is to lose weight, reduce your kcal intake by 15%. This is done by multiplying your figure by 0.85.*
- *If your goal is to gain weight, increase your kcal intake by 20%. This is done by multiplying your figure by 1.2.*

Step 5: Calculate your protein

To calculate your daily protein intake:

Multiply your lean body mass by 2.3-2.5.

The number you calculate is the recommended number of grams of protein you are advised to eat in a day.

Step 6: Calculate your fat

A good starting point for your fat intake is between 0.8-1.0g.kg.bw per day. If you prefer more fat in the diet, then go for the higher number. If you perform higher intensity, prolonged moderate/high intensity (<70%MHR) or high volume resistance training then aim for the lower range.

If your primary activity is a low volume sport such as powerlifting or Olympic weightlifting, or your goal is weight loss, then you may choose to increase your fat intake above this recommendation. This will mean that a smaller proportion of your food will come from carbohydrates.

Step 7: Calculate your carbohydrates

Carbohydrate intake is calculated by the kcals left over after working out your fat and protein needs. To do this, use the following conversions:

- Fat kcals = fat in grams × 9 (There are 9 kcals per g of fat)
- Protein kcals = protein in grams × 4 (There are 4 kcals per g of protein)
- Carbohydrate kcals = total daily kcals − fat kcals − protein kcals
- Carbohydrates in grams = carb kcals ÷ 4 (There are 4 kcals per g of carbohydrates)

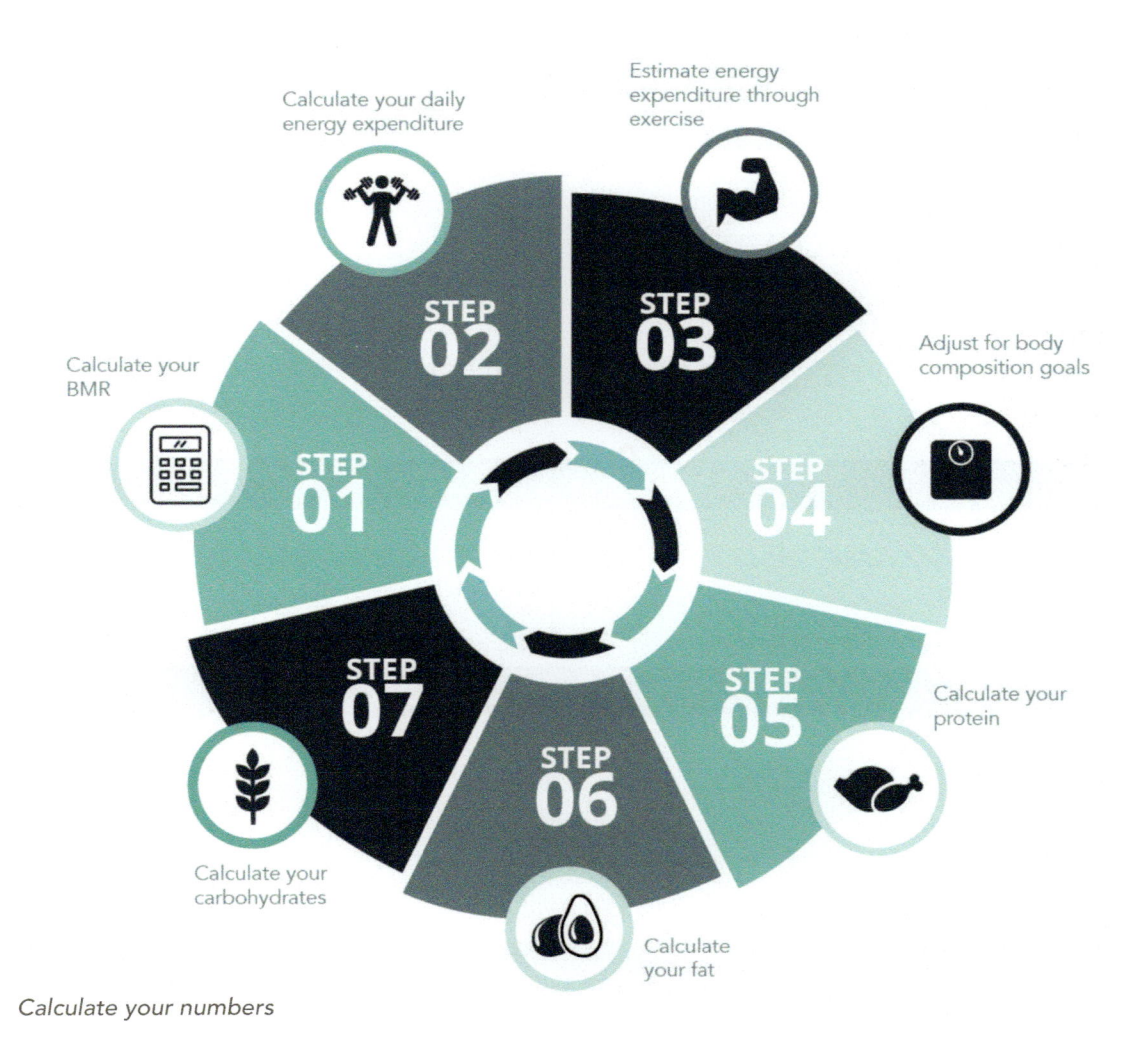

Calculate your numbers

Jonathon

Jonathon is a 30-year-old male office worker who is 180 cm tall and weighs 80 kg. Although his main goal is to put on muscle, he is also conscious that he does not want to put on any body fat.

Jonathon trains five times per week. Sessions are typically a mix of resistance training and conditioning. He also runs to work on one of these days.

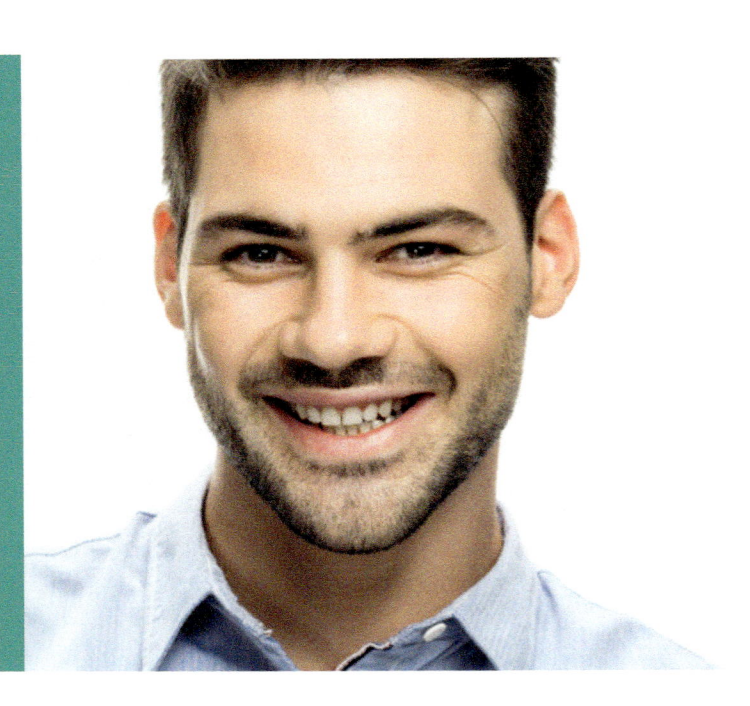

Example - Jonathon

Step 1 - Calculate BMR

Using the U.S. Navy Method body fat calculator and Katch Mcardle BMR calculation.

Body Fat (U.S. Navy Method)	
Body Fat	18.4%
Body Fat Mass	14.7 kgs
Lean Body Mass	65.3 kgs
Katch Mcardle BMR calculation = 370 + (21.6 x Lean Body Mass(kg))	
370 + (21.6 x 65.3)	1,780

Step 2 - Calculate daily energy expenditure

Jonathon has an office job, so his PAL will be 1.2 (mostly inactive or sedentary).

BMR x PAL	Adjusted for PAL
1,780 x 1.2	2,136

Step 3 - Calculate energy expenditure through exercise

Using the MET scale, it can be estimated that he expends 640 kcal for his main workouts. When he runs to work, Jonathan expends roughly an extra 300 kcals.

Based on this, his recovery or "none" workout days can be classed as a "light day", training once as a "moderate day", and days where he trains twice, as "hard days".

Exercise key	Energy Expenditure (EE)	Total Energy Expenditure (EE)
Light day	2,136	2,136
Moderate day	2,136 + 640	2,776
Hard day	2,136 + 640 + 300	3,076

Step 4 – Adjust your numbers for your goal

Jonathan's goal is improving his body composition. Therefore, we are going to start by following his maintenance numbers for 4 weeks. Based on his results (weight, body fat and change in shape) after these 4 weeks, we can look to increase or decrease his kcals.

Activity key	KCALS	Changes for weight gain
	BMR + PAL + EE	Increase your kcal intake by 20%. Multiply your maintenance calories by 1.2.
Light day	2,136	(Light day) 2136 x 1.2 = 2,563kcal
Moderate day	2,776	(Moderate day) 2776 x 1.2 = 3,331kcals
Hard day	3076,	(Hard day) = 3076 x 1.2 = 3,691kclas

Step 5 – Calculate protein intake

With Jonathon's goal being improved body composition, we will set his protein at the higher end of the scale. Multiply Lean Body Mass (LBM) by 2.5.

LBM	Protein
65.3 x 2.5	163g

Step 6 - Calculate fat intake
Jonathan prefers fattier cuts of meat and because performance is not his priority, we will set his fat number at the higher end of the scale. Multiply weight by 1.

Weight	Fat
80 x 1	80g

Step 7 – Calculate carbohydrate intake
We can calculate his carbohydrate targets by using the following formula:

Total kcals – kcals from protein – kcals from fat

	BMR + PAL + EE	Protein kcals	Fat kcals	Carbs
Light day	2,136kcal	163 x 4 = 653	80 x 9 = 720	(2,136 – 653 – 720)/4 = 191g
Moderate day	2,776kcal	163 x 4 = 653	80 x 9 = 720	(2,776 – 653 – 720)/4 = 350g
Hard day	3,076kcal	163 x 4 = 653	80 x 9 = 720	(3,076 – 653 – 720)/4 = 425g

Jonathon's starting numbers

Activity key	Kcals	Protein	Fat	Carbs
Light day	2,136kcal	163g	80g	191g
Moderate day	2,776kcal	163g	80g	350g
Hard day	3,076kcal	163g	80g	425g

Jane

Jane is a 28-year-old female who is 170 cm tall and weighs 65 kg. She also works in an office environment however, she makes a conscious effort to walk over 15,000 steps a day.

Jane trains four times per week. Three of which are weights/conditioning-based sessions and her fourth session is an hour of yoga.

Jane's goal is to lose weight.

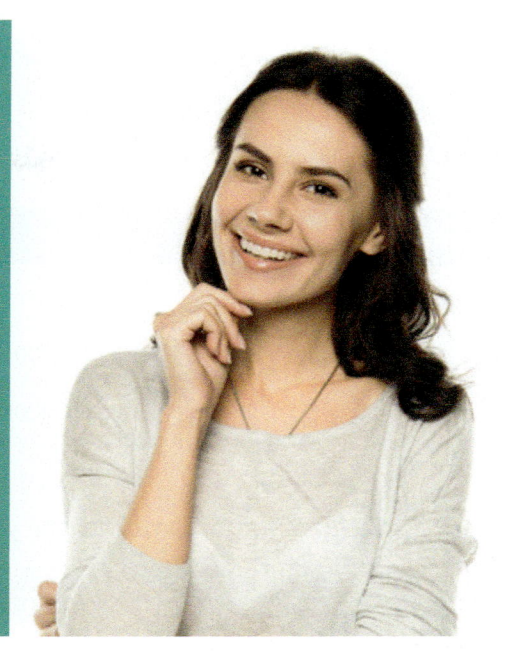

Example - Jane

Step 1 - Calculate BMR

Using the U.S. Navy Method body fat calculator and Katch Mcardle BMR calculation.

Body Fat (U.S. Navy Method)	
Body fat	26.1
Body Fat Mass	17.0kgs
Lean Body Mass	48.0kgs
Katch Mcardle BMR calculation = 370 + (21.6 x Lean Body Mass(kg))	
370 + (21.6 x 48)	1,407

Step 2 - Calculate daily energy expenditure

Because of Jane's fairly active lifestyle, we can define her PAL as 1.3

BMR x PAL	Adjusted for PAL
1407 x 1.3	1,829

Calculate Your Numbers

Step 3 - Calculate energy expenditure through exercise

Jane expends roughly 400 and 200 kcals respectively for both her weights and yoga sessions.

Exercise key	Energy Expenditure (EE)	Total Energy Expenditure (EE)
Light day	1,829	1,829
Moderate day	1,829 + 200	2,029
Hard day	1,829 + 400	2,229

Step 4 – Adjust your numbers for your goal

With Jane's goal being weight loss, we can multiply her energy expenditure by 0.85.

Activity key	Kcals	Changes for weight gain
	BMR + PAL + EE	Reduce your kcal intake by 15%. Multiply your calories by 0.85
Light day	1,829	1,554
Moderate day	2,029	1,724
Hard day	2,229	1,894

Step 5 – Calculate protein intake

As Jane's goal is improving body composition, we will set her protein at the higher end of the scale. Multiply Lean Body Mass (LBM) by 2.5.

LBM	Protein
48 x 2.5	120g

FUELLING THE FUNCTIONAL ATHLETE

Step 6 - Calculate fat intake

With Jane's goal being body composition with no specific focus on performance, we can set her fat based on her preference. As she also prefers more fat in her diet, we have set her fat at the higher end of the scale. Multiply weight by 1 to get the grams of fat.

Weight	Fat
65 x 1.0	65g

Step 7 – Calculate carbohydrate intake

We can calculate her carbohydrate targets by:

Total kcals – kcals from protein – kcals from fat

	BMR + PAL + EE	Protein kcals	Fat kcals	Carbs
Light day	1,554	480	585	(1,554-480-585)/4 = 123g
Moderate day	1,724	480	585	(1,724-480-585)/4 = 165g
Hard day	1,894	480	585	(1,894-480-585)/4 = 207g

Jane's starting numbers

Activity key	Kcals	Protein	Fat	Carbs
Light day	1,554	120g	65g	123g
Moderate day	1,724	120g	65g	165g
Hard day	1,894	120g	65g	207g

Calculate your numbers

Step 1 - Calculate BMR

Using the U.S. Navy Method body fat calculator and Katch Mcardle BMR calculation.

Body Fat (U.S. Navy Method)	
Body fat	
Body Fat Mass	
Lean Body Mass	
Katch Mcardle BMR calculation = 370 + (21.6 x Lean Body Mass(kg))	

Step 2 - Calculate daily energy expenditure

BMR x PAL	Adjusted for PAL

Step 3 - Calculate energy expenditure through exercise

Exercise key	Energy Expenditure (EE)	Total Energy Expenditure (EE)
Light day		
Moderate day		
Hard day		

Step 4 – Adjust your numbers for your goal

Activity key	Kcals	Changes for weight loss	Changes for weight gain
	BMR + PAL + EE	Reduce your kcal intake by 15%. Multiply your kcals by 0.85	Increase your kcal intake by 20%. Multiply your maintenance kcals by 1.2
Light day			
Moderate day			
Hard day			

Step 5 – Calculate protein intake

LBM	Protein

Step 6 - Calculate fat intake

Weight	Fat

Step 7 – Calculate carbohydrate intake

Step	A	B	C	D	E	F	G
Calculation				B X 4	C X 9	A - D - E	F/4
	Daily kcals	Protein (g)	Fat (g)	Protein kcals	Fat kcals	Carb kcals	Carb (g)
Light							
Moderate							
Hard							

Your starting numbers

Activity key	Kcals	Protein	Fat	Carbs
Light day				
Moderate day				
Hard day				

Any calculations and notes

8

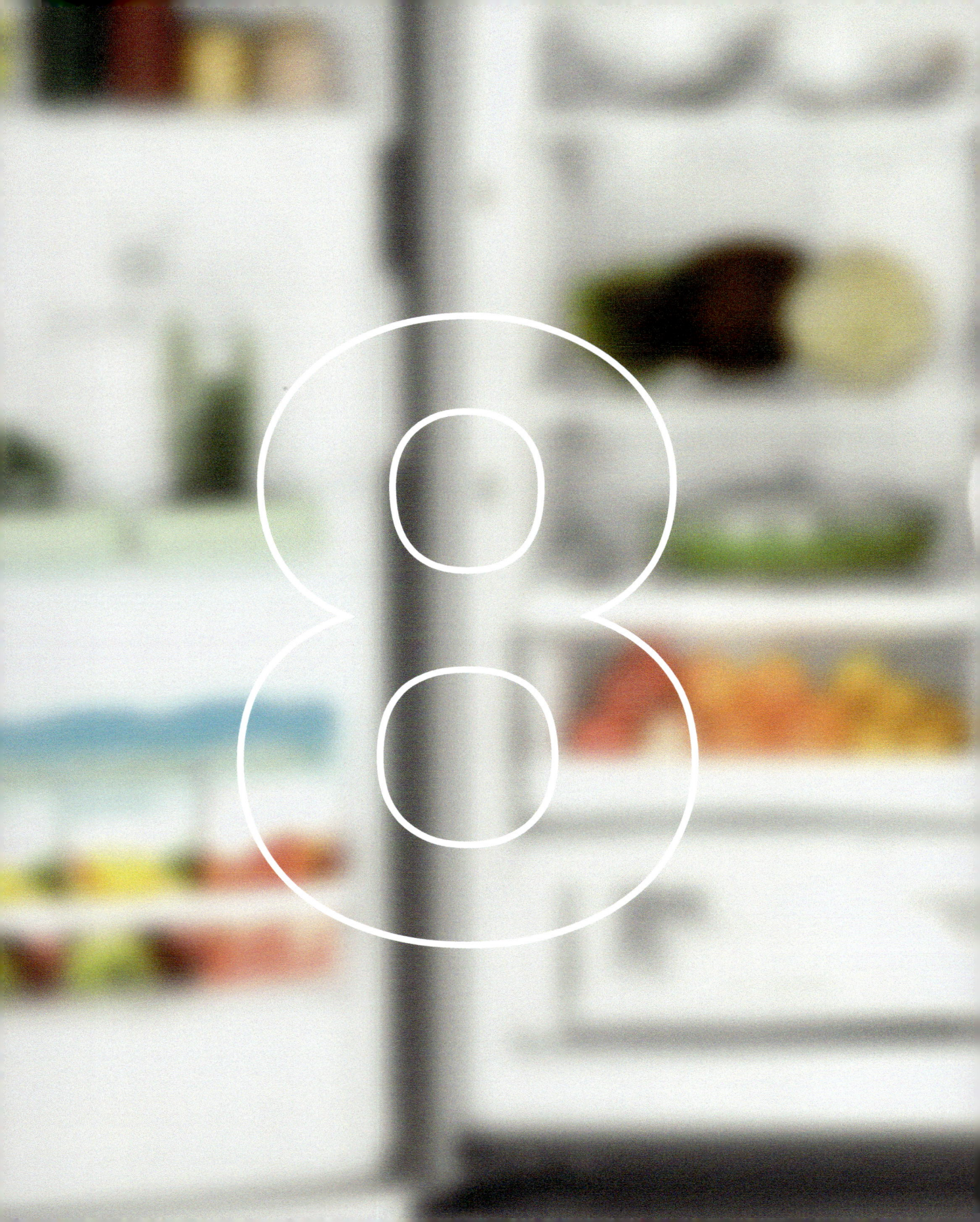

CHAPTER EIGHT

SETTING UP MYFITNESS-PAL

8.1 TRACKING YOUR FOOD

Now that you have calculated your numbers you need to plug them into a food tracking app such as MyFitnessPal (MFP).

Although some of you may be resistant to tracking, it's one of the most effective tools to improve your diet and overall habits. Writing down what you eat makes you accountable to yourself, prompting you to make better choices. A study showed that recording what you eat can actually double your fat loss efforts (18).

Tracking your food also teaches you the different values, such as the number of kcals, macronutrients and micronutrients. It also helps translate these numbers into actual foods, since, after all, we eat food not kcals! You will begin to understand foods which are carbs, fats and proteins, and how many kcals or grams of macronutrients they contain. You will learn about condiments, drinks and how to make more informed decisions in your diet and avoid sabotaging your results. This process gives you more flexibility, more knowledge and ultimately better results!

Tracking isn't something you have to do forever. In fact, at Box we encourage clients to move away from this practice and become more intuitive with their diet, however, to get to this point it pays to get a better understanding of what you're eating first. See tracking as a tool that helps you move along the continuum towards being completely intuitive, where you will not need to rely on apps such as MyFitnessPal or following a set number of kcals or macronutrients.

At Box, we follow a roadmap that focuses on low hanging fruit first, in order to see the biggest change with the least amount of effort. Adherence underpins success, which is why you want to do what you can to make your diet as unrestrictive as possible without compromising success. As your goals become more specific, so can your attention to detail with your diet.

With this in mind, we can look at the tracking tightrope. Imagine starting to walk along a wide road with plenty of room for error, where the further you take your diet, the narrower the path becomes.

Step 1- Overall kcals

The most important factor to get right whether your goal be body composition or performance, is ensuring you eat the right amount. This is why your focus should first be on overall kcals and not so much on hitting your macronutrient targets (proteins, carbs and fat). Try to aim within 100 kcals of your target.

Step 2 - Protein

Protein is arguably the most important macronutrient to prioritise. Therefore, when you feel comfortable with hitting your kcals, your next step is to focus on staying within 10g of your protein target.

N.B. It is better to be on the higher side of your protein target rather than below it. This is because protein has a higher thermic effect than carbohydrates and fat. What this means is that it requires more calories to break it down and digest. If you are likely to overshoot your calorie targets, it is more favourable that these excess calories come from protein, where it is harder to be stored as fat and be more likely to help with recovery and muscle growth.

Step 3 - Carbohydrates and fat

Once you have become comfortable with hitting your protein and kcal targets, you can start considering your fat and carbohydrate numbers. If weight loss is your goal, then you shouldn't worry about this ratio. However, if your goal is performance, we want to ensure you get enough carbohydrate to fuel any intense training and to help with recovery. Try and aim to be within 10g either side of your carbohydrate target and 5g of your fat target. The fat target is lower as fat contains more kcals per gram. Every gram of fat contains 9 kcals compared 4 per gram of carbohydrates.

Step 4 and beyond

To take things a step further, you can start looking at nutrient timings, supplement strategies, micronutrient intake, bloodwork and sugar and fat ratio. However, for most part, this is just not needed and is unlikely to bring about much change. Providing you are already focusing on the quality of your diet then the small details highlighted above are not something you should really worry about.

How to setup and use MyFitnessPal

Download and setup an account with MyFitnessPal.com.

1. Add your numbers

In custom goals, add your kcals, protein, fat and carbohydrates for the day. If you have the premium version you can change your daily targets, which are great if your training changes throughout the week. It also enables you to set targets in grams rather than percentages. Ignore the kcal burn option.

2. Focus on grams rather than the percentage

As your diet will differ from day to day based on the amount of training, using percentages to calculate your macronutrients will lead to inaccuracies. For arguments sake, if your kcals on a "none" workout day were 2000 and 30% of this will come from protein, this would be 600 kcals (150g), whereas if your kcals were 2400 on a workout day, 30% of this would be 720 kcals (180g), even though your protein target is likely to be the same day to day.

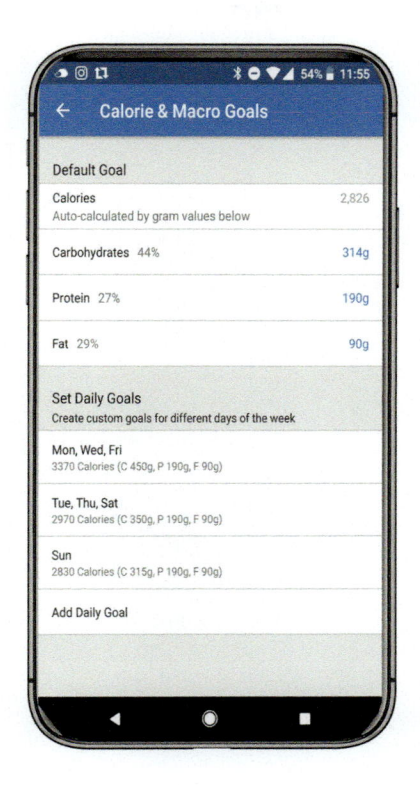

3. Track everything for a week

I know this can be tedious, but log everything for a week. Literally all that you eat and drink. So even a sip of coke, splash of olive oil or that one biscuit your colleague gave you at work. It will quickly become apparent what you're eating day to day. The more you do it, the easier it gets. By calculating your average kcals for the week, you will also be able to compare this to your average weight for the week. This gives you a solid indication of how much food you need to stay at your current weight or how to adjust it based on your goals.

Examples of foods that can quickly add up without you realising:
- *Drinks (milk, juice, soft-drinks)*
- *Dried fruit*

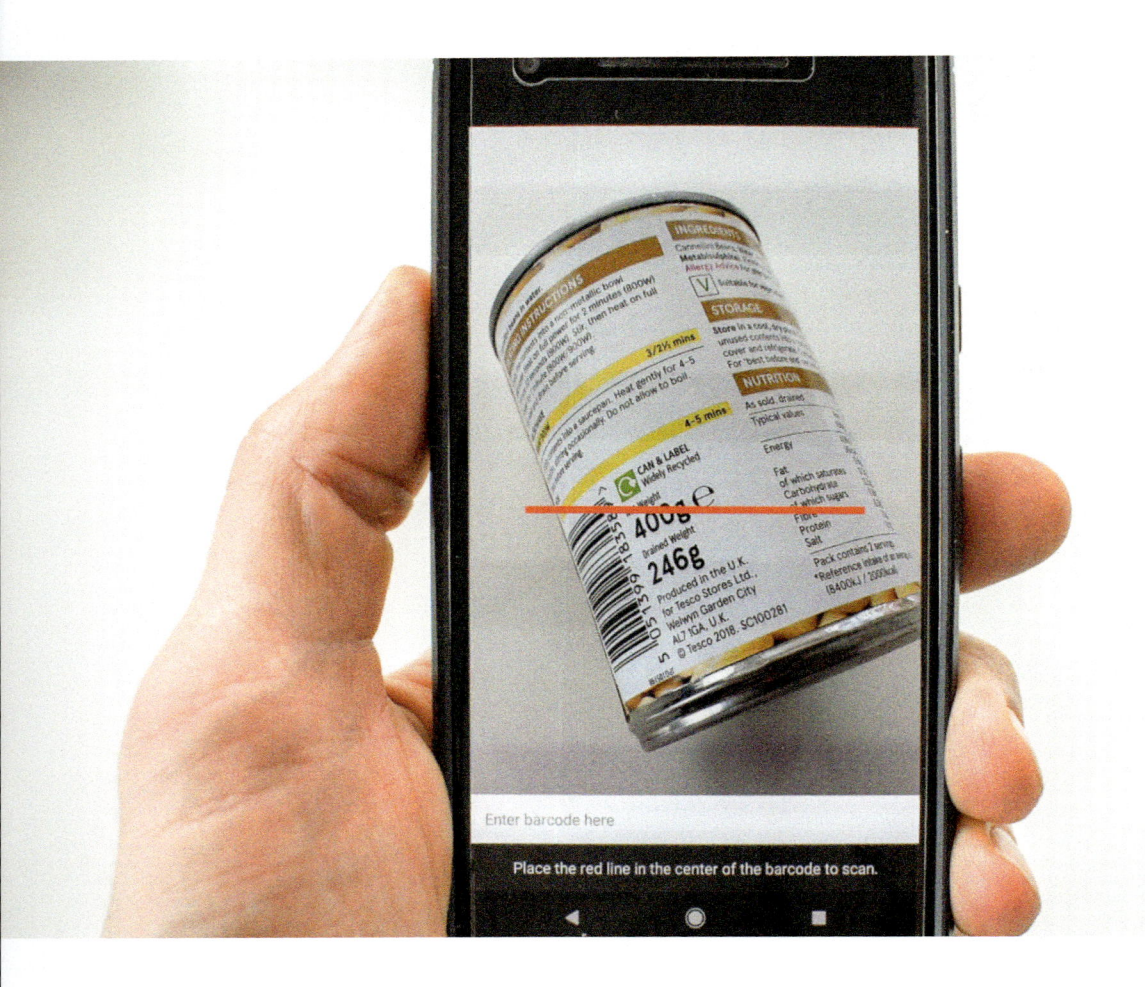

- Condiments
- Sauces
- Salad dressing
- Protein powder

4. Don't get too fixated on being exact

Kcal counting is never going to be entirely accurate. Inaccurate weighing and recording will affect this figure, not to mention how it is stored, grown and cooked. Therefore, you should simply use it as a tool to record your intake, helping paint a better picture of what changes you need to make to see improvement.

5. Don't be too inaccurate!

It sounds obvious but it's easy to wildly overestimate and underestimate your kcals, which is why we suggest you log everything for a week or two, to get a feel for it. To help you be more accurate, scan the barcode where possible, or search for the specific brand of food. Alternatively, use the search term USDA with the name of the food in your search engine. This can provide a more accurate measurement for a lot of foods.

Top tip – Buy "Carbs and Kcals" – This book is a great tool, which depicts portion sizes

---

6. Weigh your food

Do you need to weigh all your food? No, but although tedious, a small investment in time now will mean no more weighing in the future. With tracking it is important to be consistent, so either always weigh your food before you cook it (as we recommend) or after you cook it.

Top tip - Weighing from the jar – to accurately measure foods eaten from a jar, put the jar on the scales, weigh it, take out the amount you're eating and weigh the jar again.

My kcals don't add up to my macros

You may notice when tracking that even when you hit your macronutrients for the day, your kcals don't always match your targets. This is because of rounding issues with tools like MFP. There will always be an inherent error with food labelling meaning your totals for the day will not always add up. However, tracking your macros will help you hit your kcals by default so don't place too much importance on making all of your numbers match.

7. Pre-Log Your Day
Adding your food into MFP the night before gives you flexibility to ensure that what you eat fits within your targets. If it doesn't fit, then change it. This also enables you to log any future 'bad' meals, which allows you to eat around them rather than running out of space for kcals when it's too late.

8. Get reminders
Under "Settings" in MFP you can set reminders to remember to track and log your food, as you will sometimes forget.

9. Vegetables
Tracking all your green vegetables is unlikely to make a difference because of their low calorific value, whereas ignoring potatoes will. Therefore, you should create some rules when tracking your vegetables. We recommend recording starchy vegetables, which include things like potatoes, carrots, parsnips, turnips, peas and sweetcorn, whereas not to concern yourself about counting green leafy vegetables as their caloric value is inconsequential.

10. Don't forget condiments
Mayonnaise, ketchup and similar condiments are high in kcals and loaded with sugar and fat. Do not discount these when tracking.

11. Tracking on the move
If you're buying from a shop, then scan the barcode. If you're eating at a restaurant try not to worry about being too accurate as it's almost impossible. Instead, just add the protein, carbohydrate and fat source and roughly estimate its size. Once you have been tracking for a few weeks you will have a better understanding of portion sizes, making tracking on the go far easier.

12. Track alcohol

Alcohol will also skew your figures as it is not classed as a macronutrient, however it still contains a lot of kcals so it's important you track it too. What's more, you need to expend this energy first before you can start using other fuel sources. i.e. fat.

Take the kcals for alcohol you consumed from carbohydrates and fat for that day (reduce carbs and fats on days you drink alcohol).

13. Log your recipes and favourite meals

If you have similar foods for breakfast and lunch, you can save these meals into MFP and easily add them to other days.

Remember, tracking is just a tool to help you progress. The numbers you have calculated are only a starting point. Your nutrition must be fluid when using metrics like body weight, body fat percentage, circumferential measurements, gym performance, sleep and recovery time and will enable you to adjust your eating moving forward.

CHAPTER NINE

WRITING YOUR MEAL PLAN

9

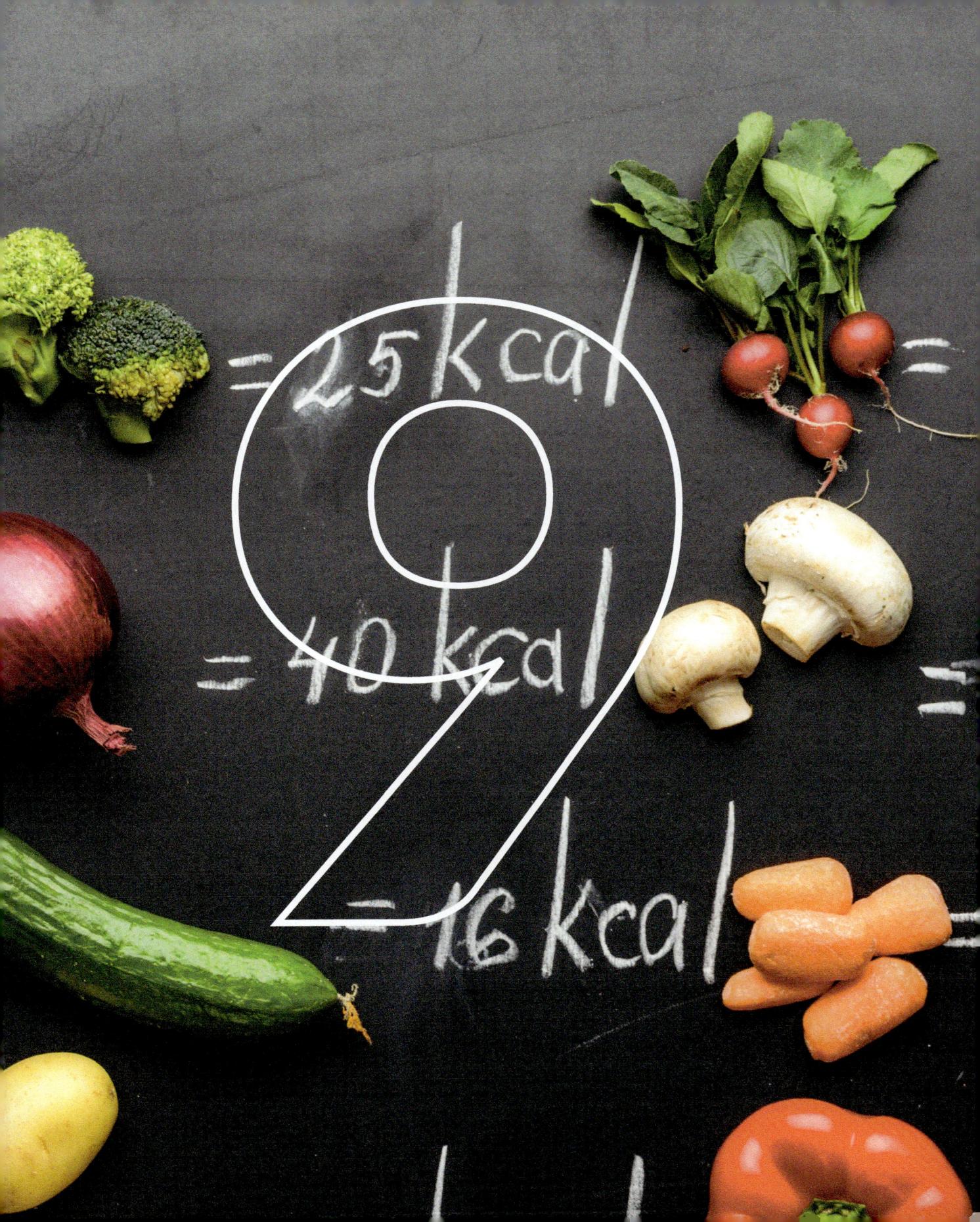

= 25 kcal

= 40 kcal

= 16 kcal

9.1 WRITING YOUR PLAN

We eat food, not kcal numbers and macro percentages, where sometimes it's this translation from numbers into a practical meal plan that can prove difficult. The following chapter goes through the framework we use to help clients build their meals and which helps to ensure you're eating the right way.

Your meal schedule

Your overall caloric intake over a 24 hour period considerably outweighs the importance of timing. That is why your personal preference and your work/social schedule should form the basis of when you eat and how many meals you eat per day. This is the reason we recommend that you only plan your main meals and workout nutrition, where the remainder of your kcals and macros can be used however you choose.

Building your meals

When building your meals, you should look to balance them by including protein, carbohydrates, fat, fruit, vegetables, condiments and fluid.

Protein

As mentioned in the protein section, to help build and repair muscle, you should ideally aim to have around 0.25-0.3g.kg.bw (around 25-40g) interspersed throughout the day, and a similar dose (0.3g.kg.bw) after exercise. Although this doesn't need to be exact (overall protein matters most), it gives us a basis to help work out your targets. You may also wish to have a larger bolus of protein before bed (0.6g.kg BW) although not essential.

Steps

1. Calculate your post workout protein serving. 0.5g x bodyweight (kg)
2. Divide the remaining protein by the amount of meals and snacks in your schedule (not including the post workout serving).

Example - 80kg athlete eating 6 meals and snacks per day

BW x 0.5	Post workout	Remaining	Per meal/snack
80 x 0.5	40g	163-40 = 123	123/5 = 24.6g

Based on your schedule, you may prefer three larger servings with your main meals and a smaller serving with your snacks. This is perfectly acceptable. The figure below depicts our protein portion size recommendations.

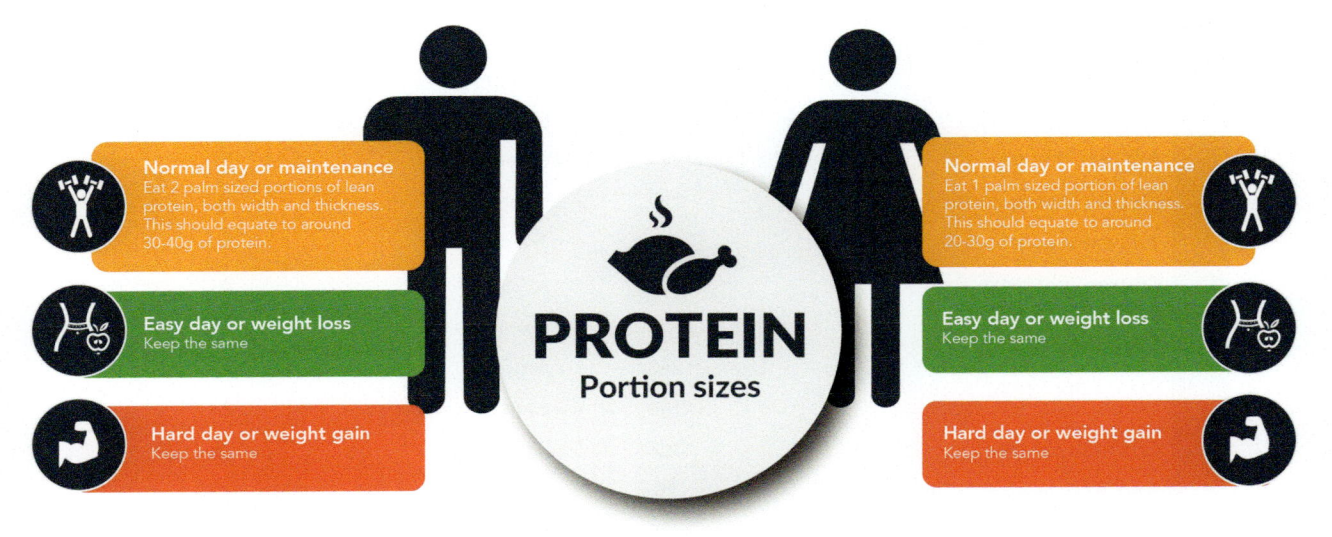

PROTEIN Portion sizes

Men:
- **Normal day or maintenance**: Eat 2 palm sized portions of lean protein, both width and thickness. This should equate to around 30-40g of protein.
- **Easy day or weight loss**: Keep the same
- **Hard day or weight gain**: Keep the same

Women:
- **Normal day or maintenance**: Eat 1 palm sized portion of lean protein, both width and thickness. This should equate to around 20-30g of protein.
- **Easy day or weight loss**: Keep the same
- **Hard day or weight gain**: Keep the same

Sources

The following table compares the kcal and macro breakdown of various protein sources.

Green foods are lower in kcals and fat. These are better choices when weight loss is the goal and for days and meals that need to be lower kcal.

Orange protein sources are moderate in kcals per serving and typically contain a moderate amount of fat.

Red denotes foods that are high in kcals and in fat. Use these sources with caution unless weight gain is the goal.

N.B. Although salmon and mackerel are high in kcals and fat, they are still a fantastic source of omega 3, which has many health benefits. Just account for the fat content when building your meals.

Food source	Quantity (g)	Serving size	Protein (g)
Eggs (chicken)	160	5 x average egg	17
Yogurt greek plain 0% fat	150	1 x larger pot	16
Turkey rashers	100	4 x rashers	21
Chicken slices	80	2 x average portion	19
Turkey slices	80	2 x average portion	18
Arla Skyr Natural	150	1 x average pot	17
Chicken Sausages (Heck)	120	2 x sausages	19
Tofu raw regular	125	1 x 1/2 cup	10
Chicken light meat raw	100	1 x small fillet	24
Arla Skyr Strawberry	150	1 x average pot	14
Prawns king raw	140	1 x cup	25
Venison meat only raw	104	4 x carpaccio slice	23
Cod flesh only raw	108	1 x medium fillet	26
Beef slices sandwich meat	80	4 x standard slice	20
Quark	150	0.6 x small tub	22
Whey protein powder	30	1 x average serving/scoop	27
Milk semi-skimmed pasteurised average	568	1 x pint	20
Beef biltong	40	1 x serving	23

Food source	Quantity (g)	Serving size	Protein (g)
Tuna canned in brine drained	130	1 x standard can (180g)	32
Turkey breast fillet grilled meat only	100	3 x medium slice	35
Turkey mince raw 2% fat	140	0.6 x small pack	34
Sea bass flesh only baked	110	1 x medium fillet	26
Minced beef 5%	140	1 x medium	29
Tinned mackerel in tomato sauce	125	1 x average can	16
Beef mince raw extra lean	140	1 x medium	31
Lamb loin joint roasted lean	90	1 x medium portion	25
Yogurt Greek style plain	150	1 x larger pot	9
Tuna canned in sunflower oil drained	130	1 x standard can (180g)	33
Chicken drumsticks	180	1 x average portion	29
Bacon rashers back grilled	75	3 x piece average	17
Beef sirloin steak raw lean	160	1 x medium	38
Turkey mince raw 7% fat	140	0.6 x small pack	32
Eggs chicken whole raw	171	3 x average	22
Salmon baked	120	1 x average portion	28
Minced beef 12%	140	1 x medium	29
Lamb mince raw	140	1 x medium	27
Mackerel flesh only grilled	125	1 x medium fillet	27
Minced Beef 15%	140	1 x medium	28
97% Pork Sausage,	120	2 x sausages	28
Beef fillet steak grilled lean and fat	172	0.8 x average 5oz	49
Chicken thigh grilled	140		32

Carbohydrates

As discussed in previous chapters of the book, we want to maximise glycogen synthesis and to help fuel and recover from your workouts. Therefore, you should aim for 1g.kg.bw after you exercise, especially if you are training again within 12hrs. We also recommend that you have another larger serving of carbohydrates before you exercise. The quantity will depend on the length of the session and how much time you have. How you split up the remainder of your carbohydrates is up to you. The figure overleaf depicts how to alter your carbohydrate portion sizes based on your goal and activity.

Steps

Calculate your post workout carbohydrate serving. 1 x bodyweight (kg)

Like protein and fat, base the rest of your carbohydrate intake for each meal on preference. Some of you may prefer a larger amount of your carbs before bed, whereas some of you may prefer to evenly distribute them throughout the day.

Eating before training

As discussed in Chapter 3 (Fuelling Your Training), the type of session will dictate how many carbohydrates you require. Unless you are training for over 60 minutes you should not need to consider any acute fuelling strategies. If your session is above 60 minutes (of work) then aim for 1g per of bodyweight of carbohydrates before you train.

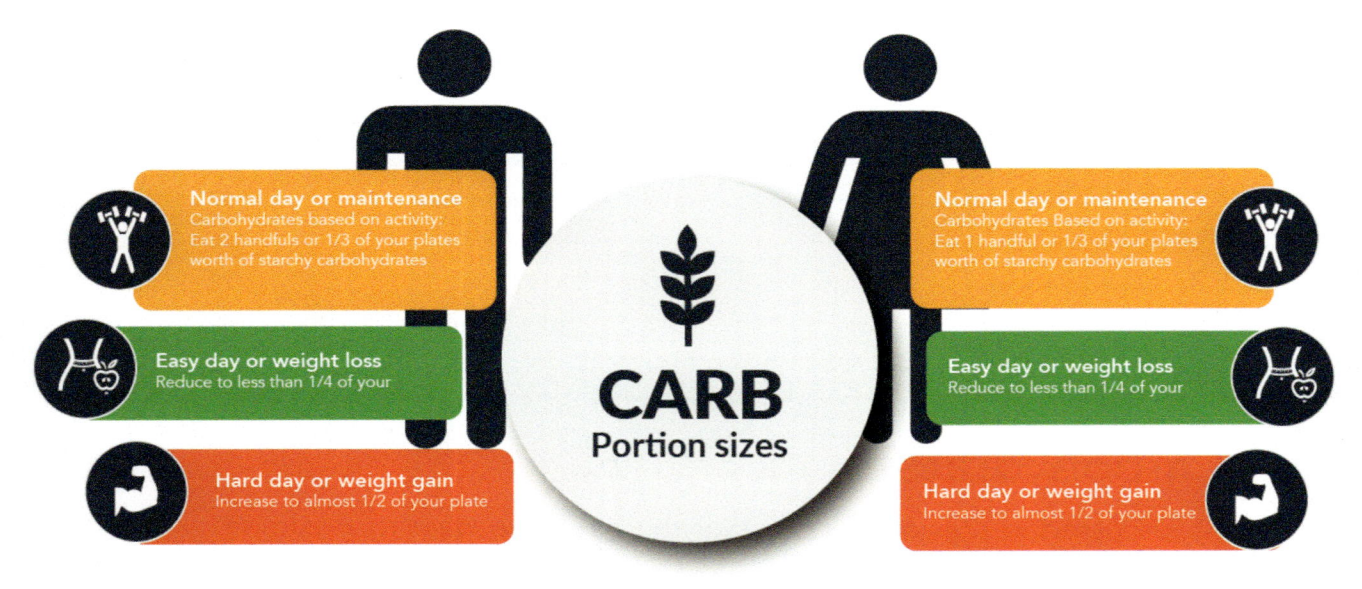

CARB Portion sizes

Men:
- **Normal day or maintenance** — Carbohydrates based on activity: Eat 2 handfuls or 1/3 of your plates worth of starchy carbohydrates
- **Easy day or weight loss** — Reduce to less than 1/4 of your
- **Hard day or weight gain** — Increase to almost 1/2 of your plate

Women:
- **Normal day or maintenance** — Carbohydrates Based on activity: Eat 1 handful or 1/3 of your plates worth of starchy carbohydrates
- **Easy day or weight loss** — Reduce to less than 1/4 of your
- **Hard day or weight gain** — Increase to almost 1/2 of your plate

Sources

It is recommended you consume mostly complex carbohydrates which are high in fibre (wholegrains, vegetables and fruit) for health benefits. These are denoted by the **lighter orange** and **yellow**. The **darker orange** represents higher kcal carbohydrates.

Starchy carbohydrates and grains

Food source	Quantity (g)	Serving size	Kcals	Carbs (g)
Carrots raw	67	1 x medium carrot	24	5
Rice cakes plain low salt	18	1 x average portion	63	13
Parsnips raw	170	1 x large portion	109	20
Sweet potato raw flesh only	135	1 x small 5"long	117	27
Breakfast cereal wheat biscuits	37	1 x average portion	120	25
Potatoes new and salad flesh only raw	200	2 x average	133	30
Oat flakes rolled	40	1 x serving 1/2 cup	149	26
Bread brown average	74	2 x medium slice	150	28
Potatoes old baked flesh and skin	165	1 x medium	156	34
Muesli Swiss style no added sugar	50	1 x average portion	177	33
Bread malt fruited	72	3 x slice	206	42
Bagel wholemeal toasted	76	1 x average portion	211	39
Rice white basmati raw	65	1 x serving	222	49
Rice brown wholegrain raw	65	1 x serving	223	46
Belvita fruit and fibre	50	1 x pack	223	34
Bagel cinnamon and raisin	82	1 x average portion	227	45
Rice cake dark chocolate	50	3 x rice cake	235	28
Granola	50	1/2 x cup (1 serving)	246	23
Banana bread homemade	80	2 x average slice	268	41
Pasta white dried	95	1 x cup	321	65
Flapjacks retail	80	1 x flapjack	348	42

Beans and lentils are carbohydrates that are also good sources of protein and fibre

Food source	Quantity (g)	Serving size	Kcals	Carbs (g)
Black beans canned drained	150	1x cup	134	19
Quinoa red and white raw	90	1/2x cup	275	46
Mixed lentils	206	1x cup	212	32
Mixed beans canned drained	150	1x cup	155	24

When carbohydrate needs are high, like for sustained sessions >90 minutes, or if training twice a day, it can be very difficult to consume sufficient amounts of complex carbohydrates. In these cases it is preferable to consume concentrated sources, such as juices, carb powders, carb drinks or sugary foods like the **red** sources listed overleaf.

Writing Your Meal Plan

Concentrated carbohydrate sources				
Food source	Quantity (g)	Serving size	Kcals	Carbs (g)
Fruit gums/jellies	30	1 x average	100	23
Fruit juice mixed	160	1 x average glass	68	17
Lucozade sport energy gel	45	1 x sachet	113	28
Maltodextrin	50	1 x 50g	188	47
Sports drink	500	1 x bottle	126	32
Vitargo powder	75	1 x serving/sachet	273	68

Fat

The timing of your fat intake does not matter so it's entirely up to you how you split up your fat throughout the day. Our only recommendation is that you reduce the fat content of meals and snacks before training to reduce any potential stomach complaints.

Fat can also be found in most other foods, especially with types of protein like dairy, eggs, fish and meat. You need to account for this when planning your meals. This may mean you need to reduce any added fat to your meals. To help monitor this, track your food with MyFitnessPal.

Our fat portion recommendations:

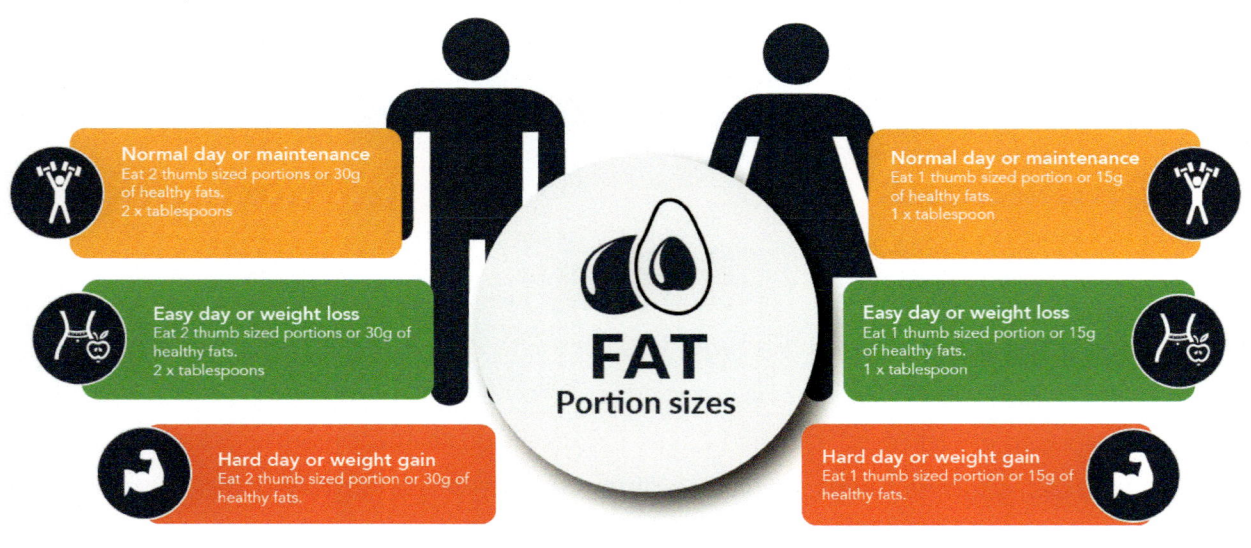

Normal day or maintenance
Eat 2 thumb sized portions or 30g of healthy fats.
2 x tablespoons

Easy day or weight loss
Eat 2 thumb sized portions or 30g of healthy fats.
2 x tablespoons

Hard day or weight gain
Eat 2 thumb sized portion or 30g of healthy fats.

Normal day or maintenance
Eat 1 thumb sized portion or 15g of healthy fats.
1 x tablespoon

Easy day or weight loss
Eat 1 thumb sized portion or 15g of healthy fats.
1 x tablespoon

Hard day or weight gain
Eat 1 thumb sized portion or 15g of healthy fats.

FAT Portion sizes

Sources

Fat

Food source	Quantity (g)	Serving size	Kcals	Protein (g)	Fat (g)
Olives	15	1 x average portion	15	0	2
Chia seeds	10	1 x tablespoon	39	2	3
Flax Seed (milled or whole)	9	1 x tablespoon (milled)	46	2	4
Almonds with skin	10	1 x average portion	58	2	5
Butter salted	14.8	1 x tablespoon	110	0	12
Oil olive	12.6	1 x tablespoon	113	0	13
Ghee butter	14	1 x tablespoon	123	0	14
Lard	14	1 x tablespoon	125	0	14
Cashew nuts kernel only plain	22	1 x average portion	126	4	11
Avocado average flesh only	70	1 x serving (1/2 Avocado)	133	1	14
Coconut flesh only fresh	45	1x piece (5x5x1cm)	158	1	16
Brazil nuts kernel only	26	1 x average portion	177	4	18
Macadamia nuts unsalted	25	1 x average portion	187	2	19
Mixed nuts (no peanuts)	30	1 x average portion	189	5	18
Oil coconut	27	1 x tablespoon (solid)	243	0	27

Fatty protein

Food source	Quantity (g)	Serving size	Kcals	Protein (g)	Fat (g)
Cheese Feta	30	1 x 5 1cm cubes	75	5	6
Cheese cottage plain	100	1 x average serving	104	9	6
Bacon rashers back grilled	50	2 x piece average	144	12	11
Beef lean average raw	121	1 x Small	156	27	5
Cheese Cheddar English	40	1 x average portion	166	10	14
Mixed nuts (no peanuts)	30	1 x average portion	189	5	18
Eggs chicken whole raw	171	3 x average size	225	22	15
Mackerel flesh only grilled	80	1 x medium fillet	226	16	18
Salmon baked	120	1 x average portion	245	28	15
Beef sirloin steak	160	1 x medium	281	43	12

What about fruit and vegetables?

Both fruit and vegetables come under the category of carbohydrates. We recommend that non-starchy vegetables should form the basis of all of your main meals and that you should look to include a variety of colours. We also recommend that you consume at least 2 portions of fruit per day. This will ensure you are attaining your fibre, vitamin and micronutrient targets.

Due to the high fibre content of legumes and vegetables, we recommend you limit the amount of foods like broccoli, cauliflower, sprouts, beans, chickpeas and lentils before you exercise to avoid stomach discomfort.

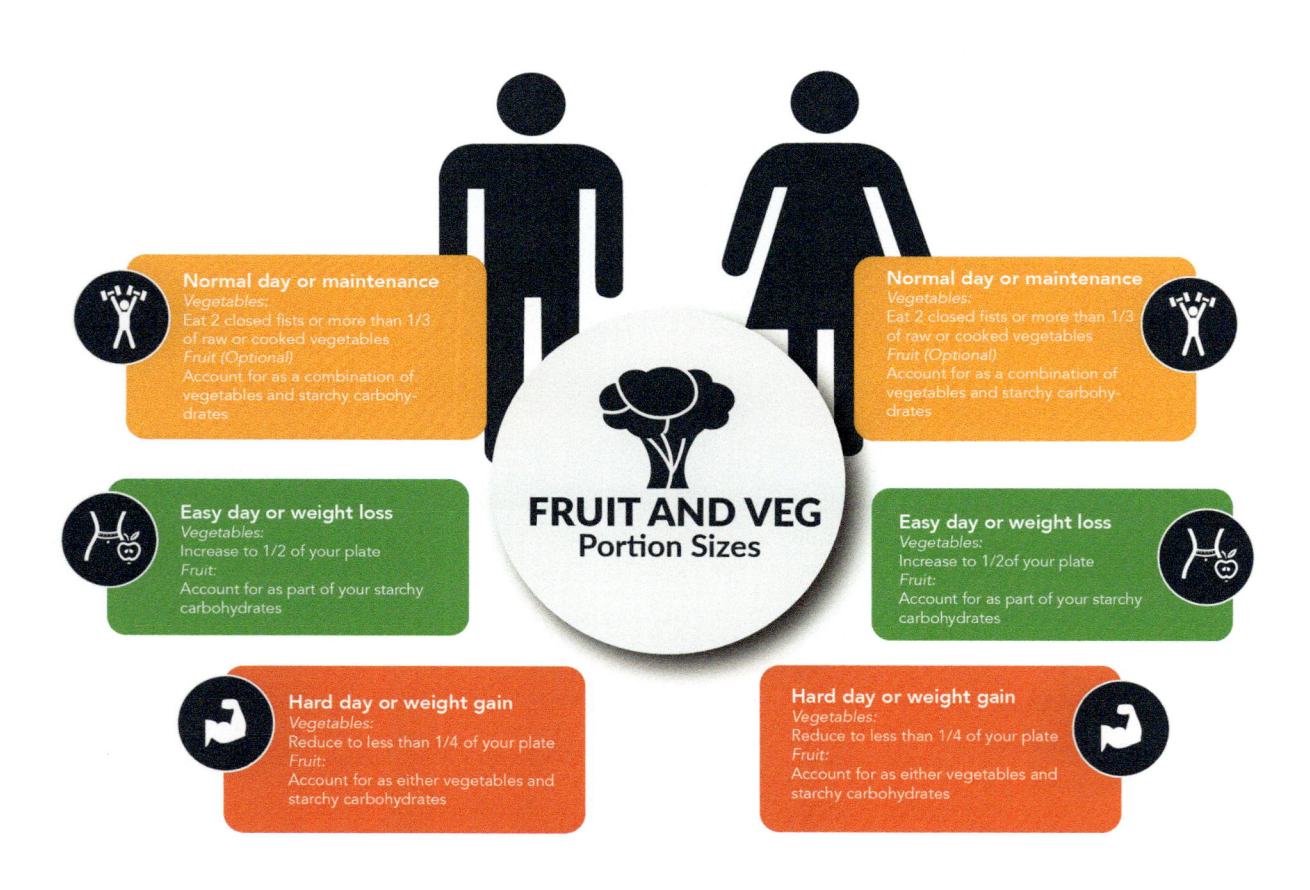

FRUIT AND VEG Portion Sizes

Normal day or maintenance
Vegetables:
Eat 2 closed fists or more than 1/3 of raw or cooked vegetables
Fruit (Optional)
Account for as a combination of vegetables and starchy carbohydrates

Easy day or weight loss
Vegetables:
Increase to 1/2 of your plate
Fruit:
Account for as part of your starchy carbohydrates

Hard day or weight gain
Vegetables:
Reduce to less than 1/4 of your plate
Fruit:
Account for as either vegetables and starchy carbohydrates

Normal day or maintenance
Vegetables:
Eat 2 closed fists or more than 1/3 of raw or cooked vegetables
Fruit (Optional)
Account for as a combination of vegetables and starchy carbohydrates

Easy day or weight loss
Vegetables:
Increase to 1/2 of your plate
Fruit:
Account for as part of your starchy carbohydrates

Hard day or weight gain
Vegetables:
Reduce to less than 1/4 of your plate
Fruit:
Account for as either vegetables and starchy carbohydrates

Eat the rainbow

Red fruits and vegetables contain lycopene, which is a pigment that gives their red colour. It is also a powerful antioxidant that may help protect the body from various ailments including cancer and heart disease. Other nutrients these red fruits and vegetables include are resveratrol and vitamin C that can also provide anti-inflammatory properties. Tomatoes (including tinned), peppers, cherries, raspberries, red apples, radishes, rhubarb, red grapes are all examples.

Blue and purple fruits and vegetables contain the pigment called anthocyanin. This nutrient has antioxidant properties that can help protect the body from cardiovascular problems and oxidative damage, which can lead to various health problems including cancer, stroke and heart disease. Examples of these fruits and vegetables include aubergines, red cabbage, blueberries, blackberries, plums and prunes.

Orange and **yellow** fruits and vegetables get their colour from carotenoids. These help to convert vitamin A in the body which can help with age related ailments, immunity, skin and eye health. Citrus fruits are also high in vitamin C which helps improve immunity. Examples include carrots, sweet potatoes, apricots, mangoes, squashes, pineapple, oranges and peaches.

Green vegetables are packed with various nutrients including folate, glucosinolates and vitamins A, C and E which have a number of health benefits. These include cardiovascular protection and anti-cancer properties (19).

Sources

Fruits				
Food source	Quantity (g)	Serving size	Kcals	Carbs (g)
Raspberries	100		27	5
Orange	100	0.5 x medium orange	28	6
Strawberries	100		31	6
Peaches raw flesh and skin	100	1.4 x small	35	7
Plums average raw flesh and skin	100	2.5 x small	38	9

Food source	Quantity (g)	Serving size	Kcals	Carbs (g)
Nectarines	100	1.4 x small	41	9
Blueberries	100	4.2 x average portion	42	9
Pears	100	0.9 x small	45	11
Apples	100	5 x slice (1/8th apple)	53	12
Mangoes	100	2.5x slice	59	14
Grapes	100	1 x small bunch	69	16
Bananas flesh only	100	1 x medium	86	20

Vegetables

Food source	Quantity (g)	Serving size	Kcals	Carbs (g)
Aubergine raw	80	0.3 x aubergine	13	2
Brussels sprouts boiled in unsalted water	80	3.8 x average	30	3
Cabbage raw	80	1 x NHS serving (1 cup shredded)	9	1
Cauliflower boiled in unsalted water	80	1 x NHS serving	24	3
Celery raw	80	1.3 x full length stick	6	1
Chard Swiss raw	80	2.2 x cup	16	2
Courgette raw	80	1 x medium portion / NHS Serving	14	1
Cucumber raw flesh and skin	80	1.5 x 1/2 cup slices	11	1
Curly kale raw	80	4.4 x cup	27	1
Leeks raw	80	1 x NHS serving	18	2
Lettuce average raw	80	1 x NHS serving (1 cereal bowl)	9	1
Mushrooms white raw	80	5 x average	6	0
Onions raw	80	4 x average portion	29	6
Peppers bell raw mixed	80	1 x NHS serving (1/2 pepper)	21	4
Radish red raw flesh and skin	80	4 x all sizes radish	10	2
Spinach baby raw	80	1 x NHS Serving (1 cereal bowl)	13	0
Tomatoes standard raw	80	1.6 x average portion	12	2
Watercress raw	80	1 x NHS Serving (1 cereal bowl)	18	0

Combination foods

Unfortunately, foods often contain a combination of the different macronutrients and sometimes even all three. This is another reason why tracking your food is a great tool to help understand the differences in food values.

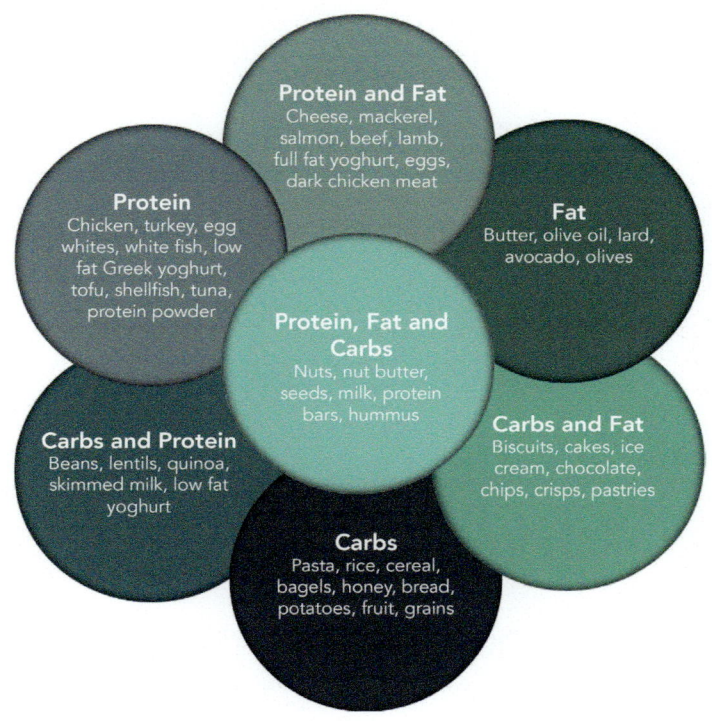

Protein and Fat
Cheese, mackerel, salmon, beef, lamb, full fat yoghurt, eggs, dark chicken meat

Protein
Chicken, turkey, egg whites, white fish, low fat Greek yoghurt, tofu, shellfish, tuna, protein powder

Fat
Butter, olive oil, lard, avocado, olives

Protein, Fat and Carbs
Nuts, nut butter, seeds, milk, protein bars, hummus

Carbs and Protein
Beans, lentils, quinoa, skimmed milk, low fat yoghurt

Carbs and Fat
Biscuits, cakes, ice cream, chocolate, chips, crisps, pastries

Carbs
Pasta, rice, cereal, bagels, honey, bread, potatoes, fruit, grains

Combination foods

Condiments

Flavour is obviously important when building your meals, however condiments like ketchup, mayonnaise and salad dressings are particularly high in kcals. This doesn't mean that you can't have them, however they need to be accounted for when tracking.

Lower kcal options include:
- *Mustard*
- *Vinegar*
- *Hot sauce*
- *Soy sauce*
- *Homemade salsa*

We recommend learning to use spices and herbs that enable you to make tasty dishes without the worry of these additional kcals.

If you are cooking	Try flavouring it with
Beef	Bay leaf, marjoram, nutmeg, onion, pepper, sage, thyme
Lamb	Curry powder, garlic, rosemary, mint
Pork	Garlic, onion, sage, pepper, oregano
Chicken	Ginger, marjoram, oregano, paprika, poultry seasoning, rosemary, sage, tarragon, thyme
Fish	Curry powder, dill, dry mustard, marjoram, paprika, pepper, fennel
Carrots	Cinnamon, cloves, dill, ginger, marjoram, nutmeg, rosemary, sage
Green Beans	Dill, curry powder, marjoram, oregano, tarragon, thyme
Greens	Onion, pepper
Potatoes	Dill, garlic, onion, paprika, parsley, sage
Squash	Cloves, curry powder, marjoram, nutmeg, rosemary, sage
Tomatoes	Basil, bay leaf, dill, marjoram, onion, oregano, parsley, pepper
Cucumber	Chives, dill, garlic, vinegar
Peas	Green pepper, mint, fresh mushrooms, onion, parsley
Rice	Chives, green pepper, onion, paprika, parsley

Drinks

As with condiments, you need to operate with some prudence when choosing drinks. If weight loss is the goal, it pays to minimise the number of kcals you get from fluid as they can quickly add up and have little effect on keeping you full. On the flip side, if your goal is weight gain then this is also the reason why liquid nutrition is a great way to help increase the number of kcals you consume.

It ultimately comes down to staying within your numbers, more so if your goal is to improve body composition. So, providing you're hitting your kcal and macronutrient targets, it's up to you how you add liquid and condiments into your meal plan.

Putting it together

Now you know what size portions are suitable for you, it's time to put your plate together. The following gives you an idea of how your main meals should look.

The following table gives you some simple examples of how to build your meals.

Meal	Protein	Fat	Carbs	Fruit and Veg	Condiments	Fluid
Breakfast	Whey	Peanut butter	Oats	Blueberries	NA	Milk
Lunch	Chicken breast	Cheddar cheese	Tortilla wrap	Spinach	Hot sauce	Water
Evening Meal	Beef strips	Olive oil	Egg noodles	Mixed veg	Soy sauce	Glass of red wine

Add your meals into MyFitnessPal

Now it's time to plug these meals into MyFitnessPal. Add in the main meals you have planned as well as your post workout nutrition. This may be part of your main meals or you may choose to add in an additional post workout snack/shake. Once you have added these meals to MyFitnessPal you may or may not have several kcals and macronutrients left over. This comes down to personal choice in how you use these kcals. You may prefer to eat more with your main meals or add in additional snacks.

After tracking for a while, you will begin to get a better understanding of how to adjust and substitute your foods and meals to meet your kcal and macronutrient goals.

Writing Your Meal Plan

Foods	Calories	Carbs (g)	Fat (g)	Protein (g)
Breakfast				
Flahavans - Oats, 50 g	188	34	3	6
Berries (mixed) - Berries (Mixed), 2 tbsp(s)	9	2	0	0
Peanut Butter, 1 tbsp	95	4	8	4
Cravendale - Semi Skimmed Milk, 150 ml	74	7	3	5
Bulkpowders - Protein, 30 gram	122	1	2	24
Lunch				
Tesco - Olive Oil, 1 Tbsp	135	0	15	0
Frank's - Original Hot Sauce, 1 tsp (5ml)	0	0	0	0
Spinach - Aldi Baby Spinach, 25 g	5	0	0	1
Sainsbury's - Wholemeal Tortilla Wraps, 1 wrap	172	28	3	6
Cheese, cheddar, 28 gram	114	0	9	7
Aladdin - Grilled Chicken Breast, 1 Each	171	0	4	32
Dinner				
Amoy - Dark Soya Sauce, 5 ml	6	1	0	0
Sainsburys - Stir Fry Veg, 100 g	27	3	0	3
Egg noodles - Egg Noodles, 1 Half pack	220	40	3	8
Tesco - Beef Strips, 100 g	120	0	4	22
Wine - Table, red, 1 glass (3.5 fl oz)	74	2	0	0
TOTAL:	1,522	122g	54g	118g

The Box Nutrition Traffic Light System

At Box, we use a traffic light system as an easy way to help you identify how to adjust your macronutrient portions depending on your goal and training. This can be used in place of tracking to help you visualise how your meals should look. Meals and days can be split up into green, orange and red.

Green Meals

Key - Easy day (none training day) or weight loss
These meals are lower in starchy carbohydrates to help reduce your kcal intake. You may choose to have once of these meals on days you don't exercise, or two if your goal is weight loss. Keep protein and vegetable intake high and ensure you are also including some healthy fats with your meals.

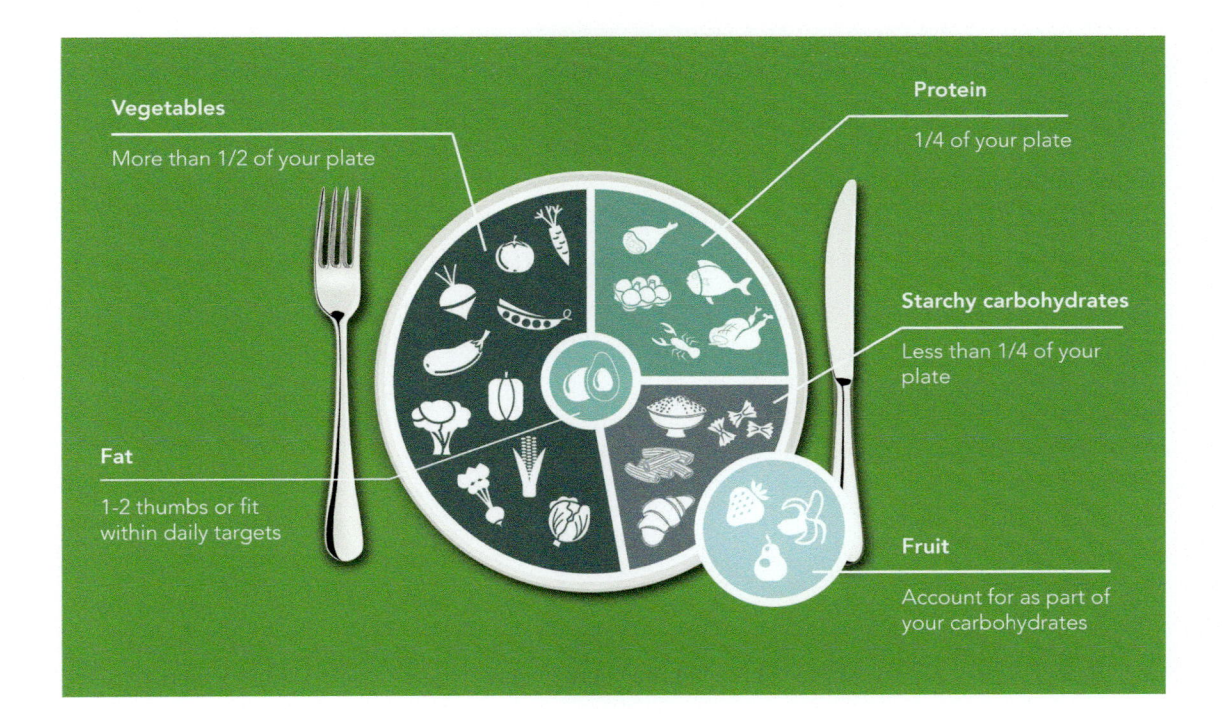

Vegetables — More than 1/2 of your plate

Protein — 1/4 of your plate

Starchy carbohydrates — Less than 1/4 of your plate

Fat — 1-2 thumbs or fit within daily targets

Fruit — Account for as part of your carbohydrates

Writing Your Meal Plan 151

Orange Meals

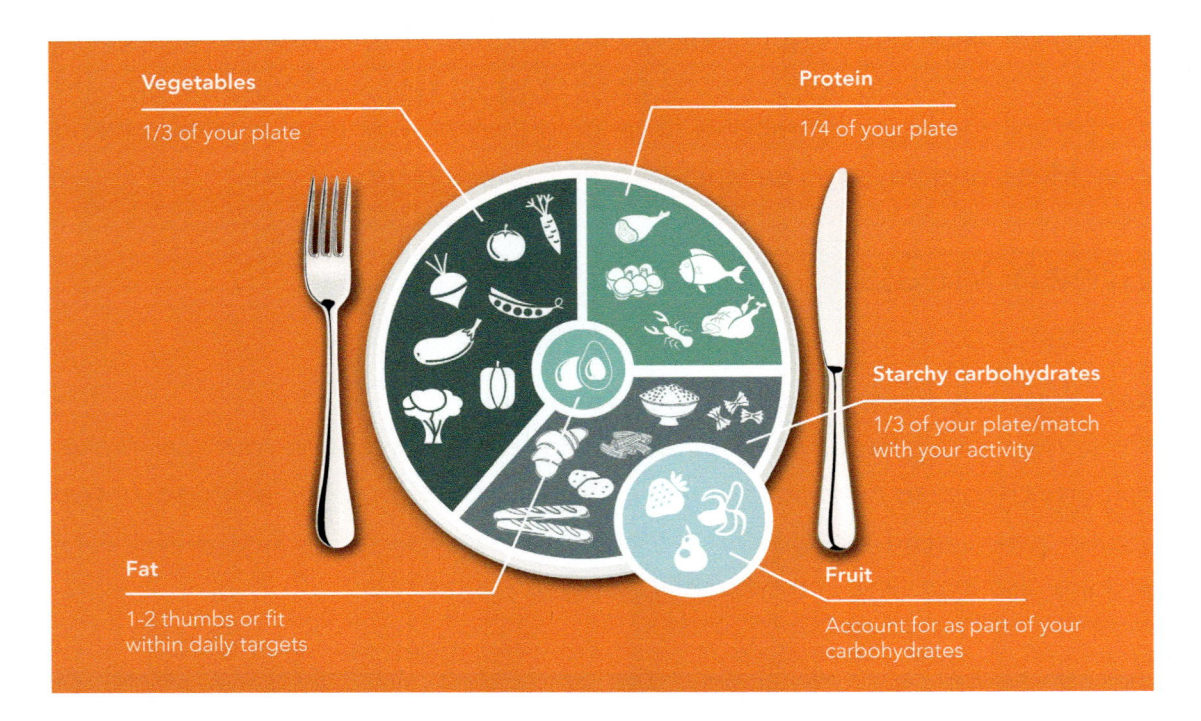

Vegetables
1/3 of your plate

Protein
1/4 of your plate

Starchy carbohydrates
1/3 of your plate/match with your activity

Fat
1-2 thumbs or fit within daily targets

Fruit
Account for as part of your carbohydrates

Key - Normal day (training once) or maintenance

These are typical balanced meals with a combination of protein, carbohydrates, vegetables and fats. The aim with orange meals is to try and match your carbohydrates with your activity level. Although this will change based on the type of activity you are performing, learn to listen to cues such as energy levels and hunger to help adjust your quantities accordingly. For example, longer more intense aerobic conditioning workouts will warrant more carbohydrates compared to a weightlifting session.

Red Meals

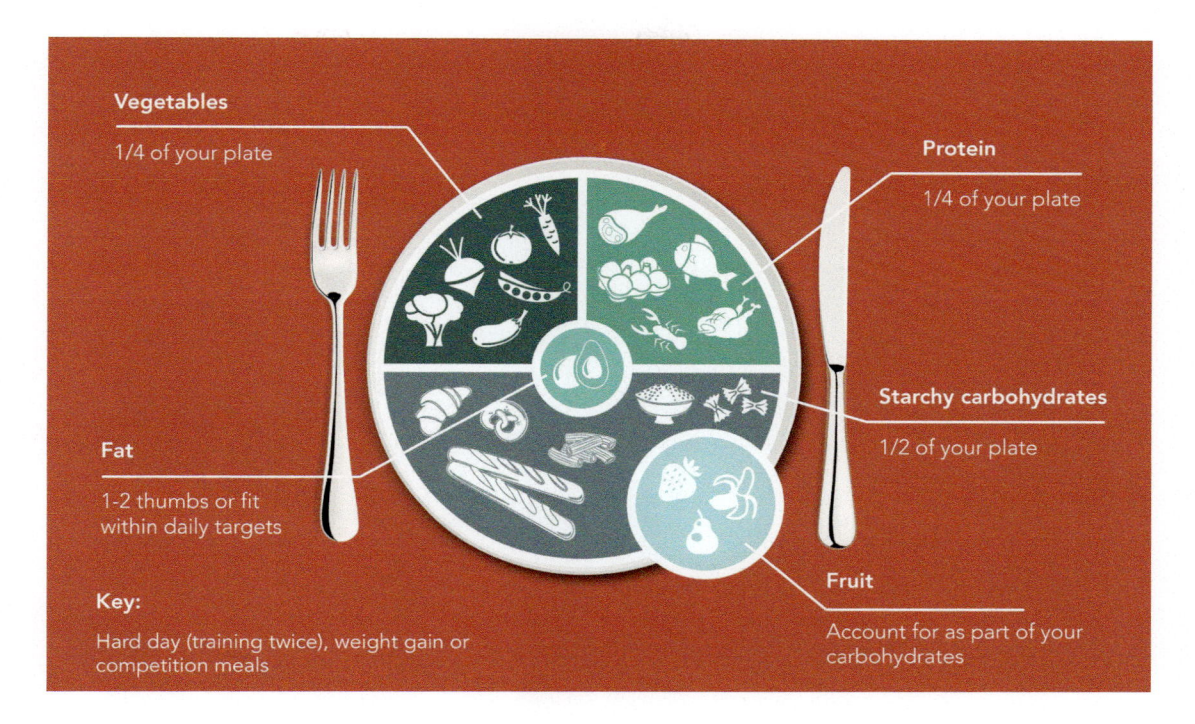

Vegetables
1/4 of your plate

Protein
1/4 of your plate

Starchy carbohydrates
1/2 of your plate

Fat
1-2 thumbs or fit within daily targets

Fruit
Account for as part of your carbohydrates

Key:
Hard day (training twice), weight gain or competition meals

Hard day (training twice), weight gain or competition meals

These are the meals and snacks used to help fuel intense or double sessions, competition and aid recovery. On these days we advise you to aim for larger carbohydrate portions and to also include 2 x carbohydrate snacks during the day.

Writing Your Meal Plan

10.

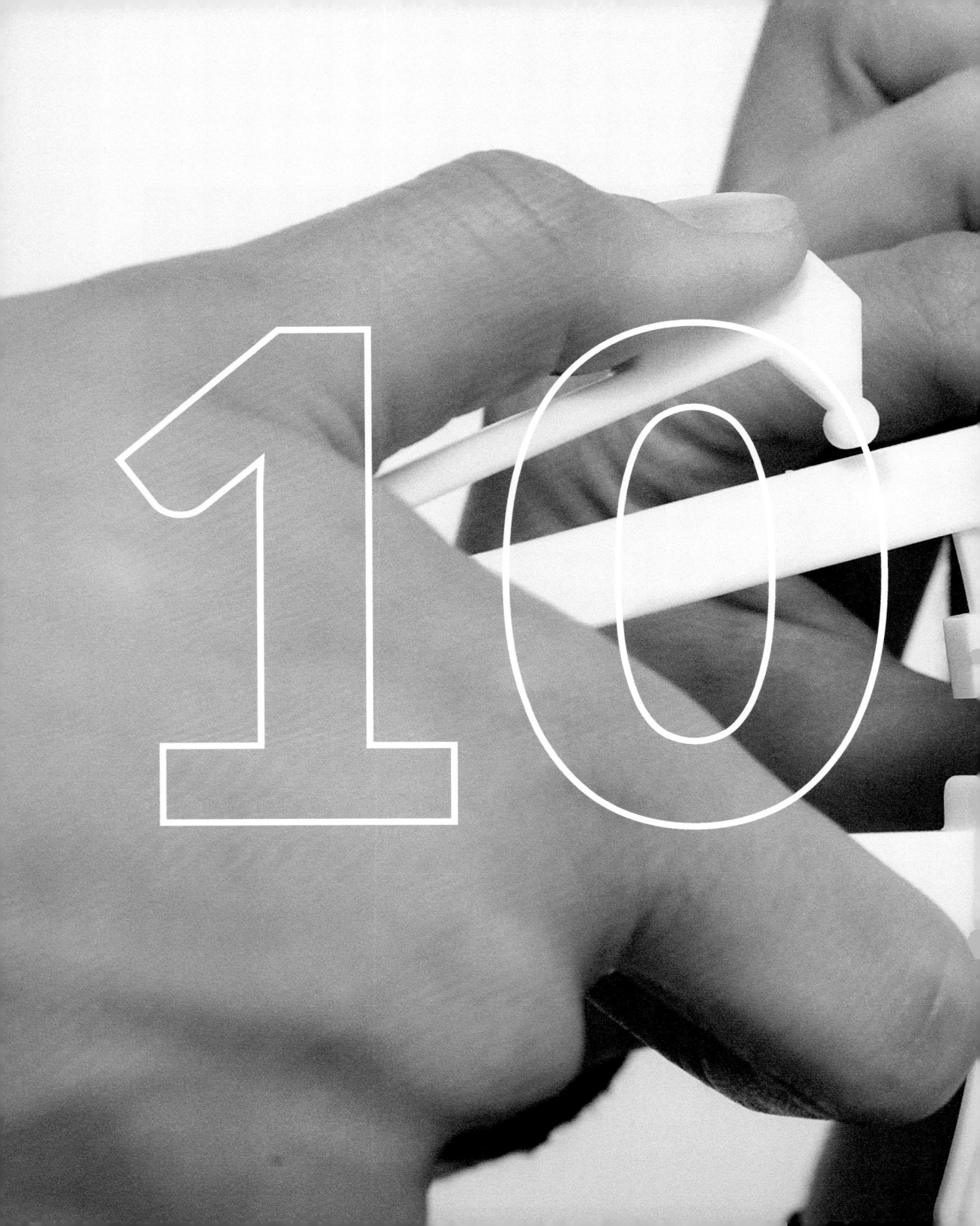

CHAPTER TEN

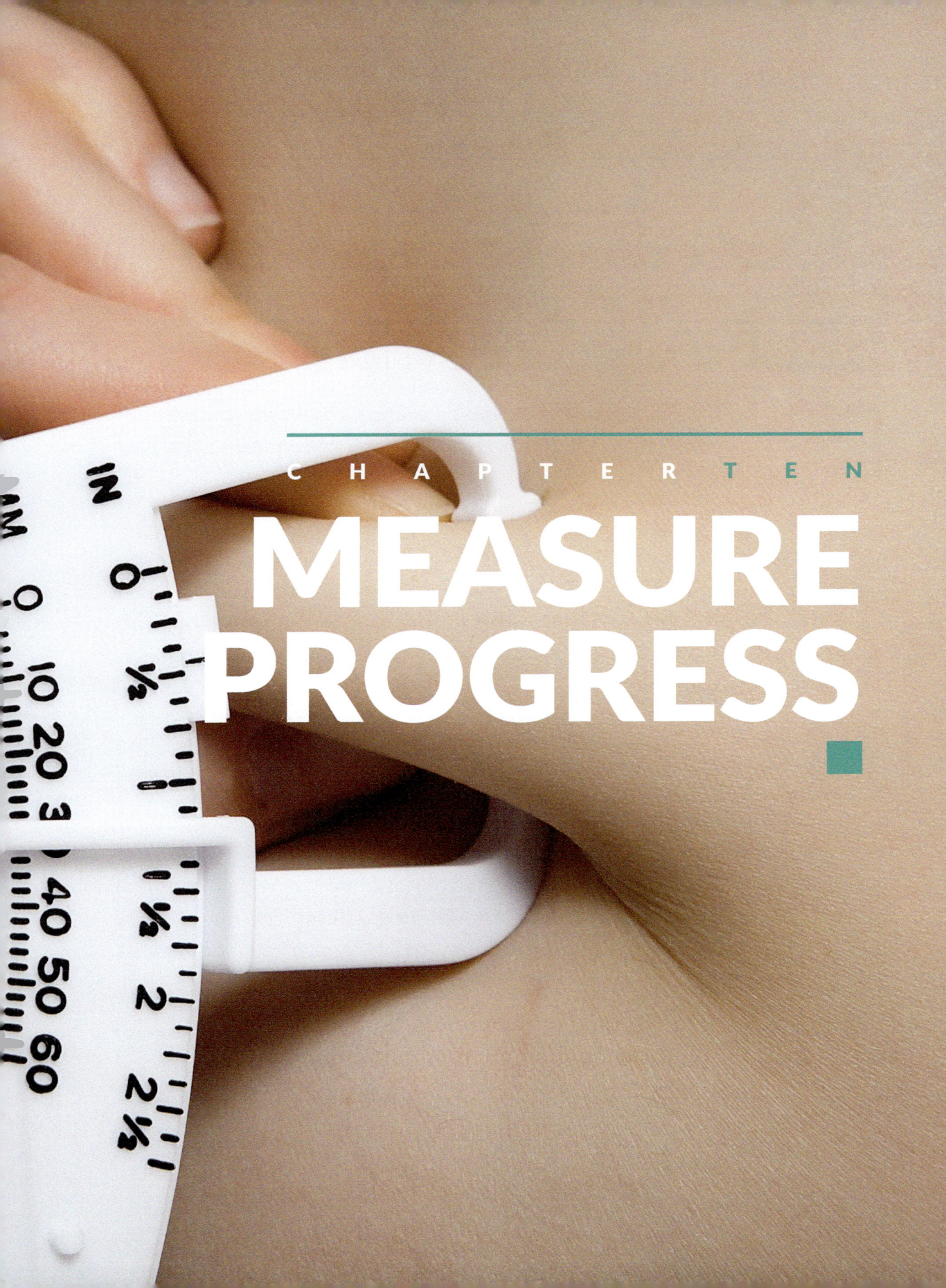

MEASURE PROGRESS

10.1 SELF-ASSESSMENT

Performing a self-assessment gives you a snapshot of where you are now, enabling you to monitor progress and acting as a good motivational tool moving forward.

Your goal will dictate which metrics to use and how often you should measure. Whether your goal is weight loss or a change in body composition, then measuring progress is more important than if your goal is to feel a little better. Don't view these behaviours as something you are required to do forever, but only a way to get back on track, reach a desired outcome and gain a better understanding of how well your diet is working.

Weight

Your weight is a simple measure to identify if you need to eat more or less. Try and weigh yourself at the same time (preferably in the morning) 3-4 times per week. At the end of each week, calculate your average by dividing the total weight by the number of days you have weighed yourself. Try not to worry about the number itself, use it only as a metric to help give you a better idea about how much you should be eating.

Although scale weight is an important metric to follow, you must be aware of some of the reasons for its fluctuations as it's not always going to be fat gain/loss.

1. *Glycogen (carbohydrates) is stored in the muscle alongside water. Based on weight, the relation of glycogen and water in the muscles will be around 1:3 in favour of water. Considering your glycogen storage can be in excess of 400g, the associated water can account for a lot of weight.*
2. *Resistance training leads to increased intracellular hydration (more water in your muscles). This will also affect scale weight.*
3. *Drinking more water will also increase hydration and the water you store in your body leading to an increase in weight.*
4. *Food in the gut, digestion rates and bowel movements (how much food passing through your body) will also impact your scale weight.*
5. *Menstrual cycle – For female athletes, water retention and an increase in body water is a common symptom during the menstrual cycle (20), particularly during the late follicular and luteal phase which may lead to weight gain (21). Sugar cravings and a reduction in energy expenditure can also lead to a fluctuation in weight during parts of your menstrual cycle.*

How to get around this

- *Take the number at face value - Use your weight as a metric of where you are now rather than a measurement of success or failure. This is only to help you adjust your kcals moving forward.*
- *Weigh often - Weighing yourself once per week can be skewed by the above factors, whereas weighing 3-4 times per week at the same time builds a more realistic image of your weight.*
- *Track your period - If you are a female athlete, track your menstrual cycle with an app like Fitrwoman to understand when fluctuations may occur.*
- *Use other metrics - Photos, body fat, how your clothes fit and circumferential measurements are just as important as weight, if not more so when your goal is a change in body composition.*

Progress photos

Progress photos helps show you changes in body composition and act as a good motivational tool. They also show us any improvements in the way we look, which, for many, is the reason to undertake a new eating regime.

Taking your photographs
1. Take photos at the start of the process and every 3- 4 weeks.
2. Wear minimal clothing
3. Set the camera up so you get an almost whole body shot
4. Take 4 photographs: front, back and both sides of your body
5. Relax when taking the pictures
6. Record these photos on your phone or in a tracking sheet provided in the resource section

Circumferential measurements

Circumferential measurements (measuring the circumference of body parts such as your waist and hip) provide another good indication of changes in your body composition and muscle mass.

Taking your measurements
Take your measurements every 2 weeks. Record them at the same time of day, preferably when you measure your weight. Consistency is key here so try and be as accurate as possible or get someone to help you.

Guidelines on how to measure
- Measure in centimetres and to the nearest millimetre
- Wear the same clothes each time. We recommend you wear minimal or tight-fitting clothing
- Breath normally
- Perform two to three measurements for each area of the body and record the average

Sites to measure
1. *Waist – around your navel*
2. *Hips – your widest part*
3. *Chest – arms up and around your nipples*
4. *Both arms – the midway point between your elbow and protruding bony part of the shoulder*
5. *Both legs – the midway point between the crease in your hip and your knee*
6. *Neck - baseline only to calculate body fat*

Body fat percentage

Your body fat percentage is the number that indicates how much of your body is made up of fat. So, if you're 85 kg and you have 15 kg of body fat, your body fat percentage is 17.6% (15/85). Knowing your body fat enables you to calculate your Lean Body Mass (LBM), which in turn helps you be more accurate when calculating kcals and macronutrients for your meal plan. Your LBM is the weight of everything in your body excluding fat. This includes muscle, organs, bones and water.

LBM is important because when calculating your kcals and macronutrients, weight alone can be misleading should your body fat percentage be relatively high. This is because muscle has a higher energy requirement than fat, meaning it burns more kcals at rest. So, if you're heavier because of a high body fat percentage rather than lean body mass, calculating your kcals off weight will overestimate your needs. If you're lean, then it doesn't matter too much.

Your protein requirements are influenced by muscle mass, so it also makes sense to calculate these by lean body mass rather than weight alone.

Body fat is a difficult metric to measure accurately unless you have access to expensive equipment like a DXA scanner or hydrostatic weighing. Bioelectrical Impedance (BIA) on your scales at home is notoriously inaccurate and it can also be difficult to find someone who is competent using skin fold callipers.

For this reason, we recommend you use the U.S. navy system to calculate your body fat percentage and lean body mass.

To do this:
1. Measure the circumference of your waist around the navel for men, and at the level with the smallest width for women. Do not suck in your stomach.
2. Measure around your neck starting below the larynx, with the tape sloping downward to the front. Avoid pushing your neck outwards.
3. For women only: Measure around the widest part of your hips.
4. Enter your results at **https://www.calculator.net/body-fat-calculator.html**

Although this may not be very accurate, it still falls within an acceptable range to help calculate your kcals and macronutrients for your meal plan.

Performance metrics

If performance is your goal, it is important to record some of your exercise metrics such as weights lifted, time or distanced covered. This will obviously be relevant to your sport or activity. If you partake in general functional fitness then write down at least one strength lift (5 rep max squat/deadlift/bench press) and one endurance workout (5k run, 2k row). Try and repeat this every 4 weeks.

Adherence

To help monitor adherence to your plan, we recommend that you note down your kcals and protein at the end of each day as well as record the average for the week. You can then cross reference this with the targets you set.

- Aim to stay within 100 kcals of your target
- Aim to stay within 10g of your protein target

You can also note down other metrics to help develop habits that stick. These could include examples like step count, days you went to the gym, number of vegetable portions you have eaten, the amount of water or alcohol units drank.

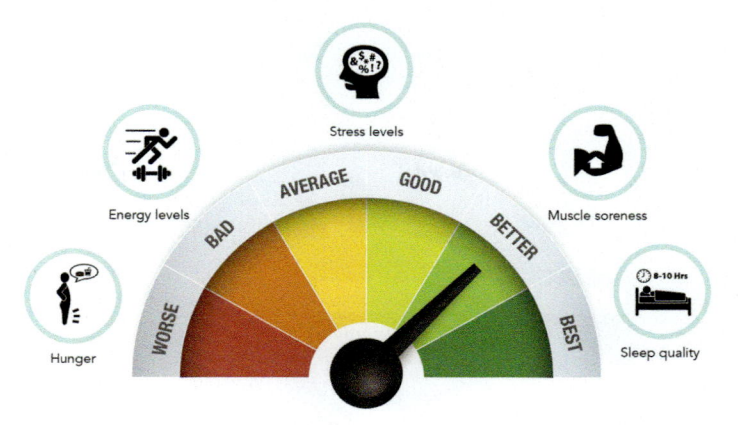

Stress levels · Energy levels · Muscle soreness · Hunger · Sleep quality (8-10 Hrs)

Worse — Bad — Average — Good — Better — Best

Your wellbeing score

As well as more objective measures like those listed above, it is also important to take note of more subjective metrics such as your wellbeing. A drop in energy levels, increase in stress, muscle soreness or poor sleep quality may indicate that you need to make changes to your nutrition, training plan or pay more attention to your personal welfare. Using a progress tracker like the one provided in the resource section, adopt a rating scale of 1-5 for each of the metrics (1 being the worst and 5 being the best).

Try and complete the wellbeing assessment every day for the first two weeks to give you an idea of how you currently feel. After a few weeks you will become aware of your 'norm', which can be used as your baseline figure. From this point, you should only need to measure your wellbeing score at the end of each week. An increase or decrease in your score will highlight areas that you will need try and improve.

Your weekly assessment

Each week you should set aside some time to complete your self-assessment. This process may seem a little arduous to begin with, however by tracking metrics like the above, you will be able to identify if progress is being made and be able to make any necessary adjustments. Remember that this is temporary and once you become more "in tune" with what you are eating, it will start to become second nature. Download your example progress tracker in the resource section provided.

CHAPTER ELEVEN
MAKING ADJUSTMENTS

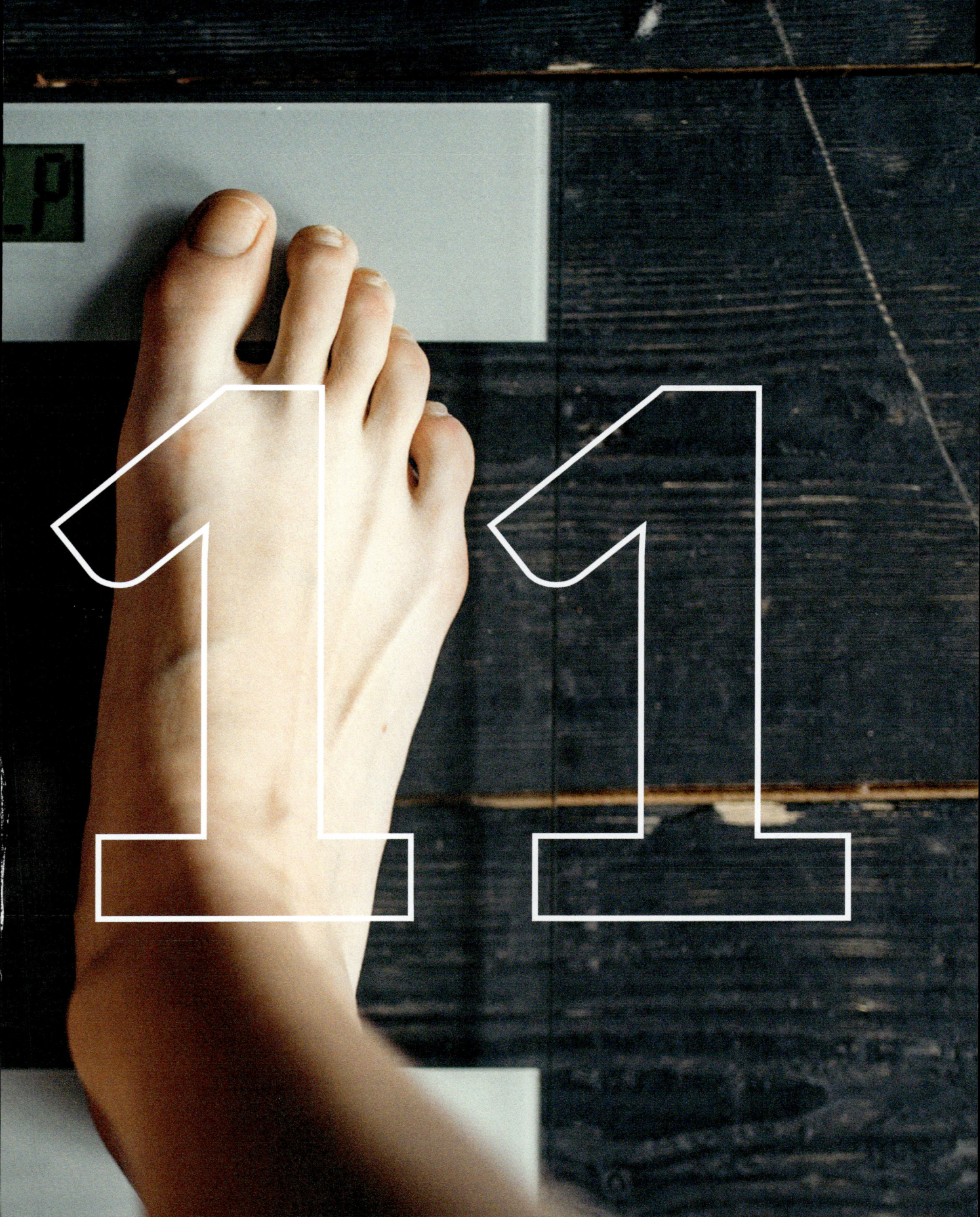

11

11.1

ADJUSTING YOUR PLAN

Once you have your starting numbers (kcals and macros) worked out, it is important to understand how to make any necessary adjustments moving forward. Unfortunately, these starting figures will never be entirely accurate considering the calculations are based on averages rather than individual differences. For this reason, you must accept that your nutrition must be fluid, whereby you must be willing to adapt your plan based on progress made.

Steps to making any adjustments

Give it time

We recommend that you spend the first four weeks just to find a setup to match your requirements. This means dieting on the highest number of kcals possible. I know this may seem counterintuitive, but it will allow you to determine whether you need to eat less or not. Who would want to if they didn't have to? Therefore, try not to make any adjustments for the first 3-4 weeks as it takes some time for the body to 'catch up' to any changes in your food intake. If you've only been following your kcals for a week or two, try and persist for another week at least.

The only exception is if you really know something isn't right and you can see that you're putting on weight or losing too much weight. In these cases, you may need to react accordingly. Such situations may be the result of over or under estimating your physical activity levels, exercise intensity or basing your nutritional values on your total weight instead of lean body mass.

If this is the case, follow the adjustment steps listed below.

1. Make sure you've been tracking

Ensure you have been tracking (weight, photos, circumferential measurement, gym performance, adherence and food) and have been consistent for 3-4 weeks, as this data will enable you to see what's happening. Although all this tracking can seem like a chore, it is exactly this practice that will ensure adherence, and thus change.

2. Look at your results

After four weeks, look back at your weight (remember to take an average for each week) and look for changes in your status or progress in photos and measurements.

If you have seen some positive changes and are heading in the right direction, keep doing what you're doing.

Weight loss targets

For weight loss we're looking for a 0.5-1% decrease in bodyweight each week. To calculate the change in percentage between weeks, work out the difference, then divide the change by the original number and multiply by 100 (see p.83 to calculate your target).

% Decrease in Bodyweight:
Week 1 = 90.1kg (Starting Weight)
Week 2 = 89.8kg

=((90.1kg-89.8kg) / 90.1kg) * 100
=0.3% Decrease

Weight gain targets

As previously discussed in expectations (p.86), weight gain will depend on your training history which can vary between a 0.5 and 1.5% increase per month.

% Increase in bodyweight = Increase ÷ Original Number × 100.

If there has been no change, or you are seeing a change for the worse, ask yourself:

1. Have you been sticking to your plan within 90% accuracy?
2. Are you struggling with sleep?
3. Are you struggling with stress?

If the answer is yes to number 1 and no to 2 and 3, you need to start making some adjustments. If it's a no to question 1, ask yourself where else you might improve and take the necessary action.

How do you make the adjustments?

For weight loss

Reduce your starting kcal intake by 5-10%. So, if your starting figure was 2500, this would mean you reduce your kcals by 125-250 kcals per day (2500*0.05=125) (2500*0.1=250). Keep protein intake on the same level. This is the macronutrient that helps keep and build muscle and helps keep us full, so it makes sense to keep this high.

Reduce your kcals from fat and carbohydrates

It does not matter too much what ratio we choose, it will come down to personal preference. I would recommend a 50:50 even split, however a higher carb diet will favour those performing at higher intensity and performing more higher repetition resistance exercise. Ensure you do not reduce fat to below 0.6g.kg.bw per day.

BW:	64		
	Non workout day		
Total kcals	1837		
	PRO	CHO	FAT
g/kg/bw	2.2	3.0	0.9
g's	141	192	56
%	31	42	28
	Moderate Day		
Total kcals	2098		
	PRO	CHO	FAT
g/kg/bw	2.2	4.0	0.9
g's	141	256	57
%	28	43	29
	Hard day		
Total kcals	2413		
	PRO	CHO	FAT
g/kg/bw	2.2	5.0	1.0
g's	141	320	63
%	23	53	24

BW:	64		
	Non workout day		
Total kcals	1745		
	PRO	CHO	FAT
g/kg/bw	2.2	2.8	0.8
g's	141	179	52
%	32	41	27
	Moderate Day		
Total kcals	1993		
	PRO	CHO	FAT
g/kg/bw	2.2	3.7	0.8
g's	141	237	54
%	28	43	29
	Hard day		
Total kcals	2292		
	PRO	CHO	FAT
g/kg/bw	2.2	4.7	0.9
g's	141	301	58
%	25	52	23

Then continue with the process of taking your measurements and photos every 2-3 weeks, and your average weight for the week. If there is still no progress, then take another 5-10% off your kcals.

For weight gain

If your goal is weight gain and you're not seeing any change, increase your kcals by 5-10%. Use the same rules as above and keep protein constant, adjust your kcals from carbs and fat and ensure you keep your daily fat targets above 0.6g.kg.bw per day.

Making the switch from fat loss to building muscle

To transition from a fat loss to a muscle gain phase, you should only increase your kcals up to your maintenance level (how many kcals you require to stay at the same weight) to prevent any unwanted fat gain. This would equate to an increase of around 15-20% or 300-600 kcals. Follow these maintenance kcals for 3-4 weeks before increasing your kcals again using the same adjustment method mentioned above (5-10% each month). Lean individuals or those who have a high NEAT (high daily activity) may benefit from a larger and more aggressive kcal surplus.

Switching from weight gain to a fat loss phase

To move from a weight gain to a fat loss phase, we also recommend that you follow a maintenance period for at least 2 weeks between phases. This is to help reduce the chances of losing muscle mass. To do this, decrease your kcals by 10% from carbohydrates and fat. After this maintenance phase, multiply your kcals by 0.85 to get your starting numbers for your fat loss phase. Like with any other stages of the diet, track weight and other metrics aforementioned to determine any further changes that maybe necessary.

To sum up

- Weight loss - Decrease your starting kcal intake by 5-10% if you're not losing weight after 3-4 weeks. Take these kcals from carbohydrates and fat

- Weight gain - Increase your kcals by 5-10% if you're not gaining weight after 4 weeks. Add these kcals to carbohydrates and fat

- When transitioning from a weight loss phase to a weight gain phase, follow a maintenance phase for at least 3 weeks

- When transitioning from a weight gain phase to a weight loss phase, follow a maintenance phase for at least 2 weeks

1.2

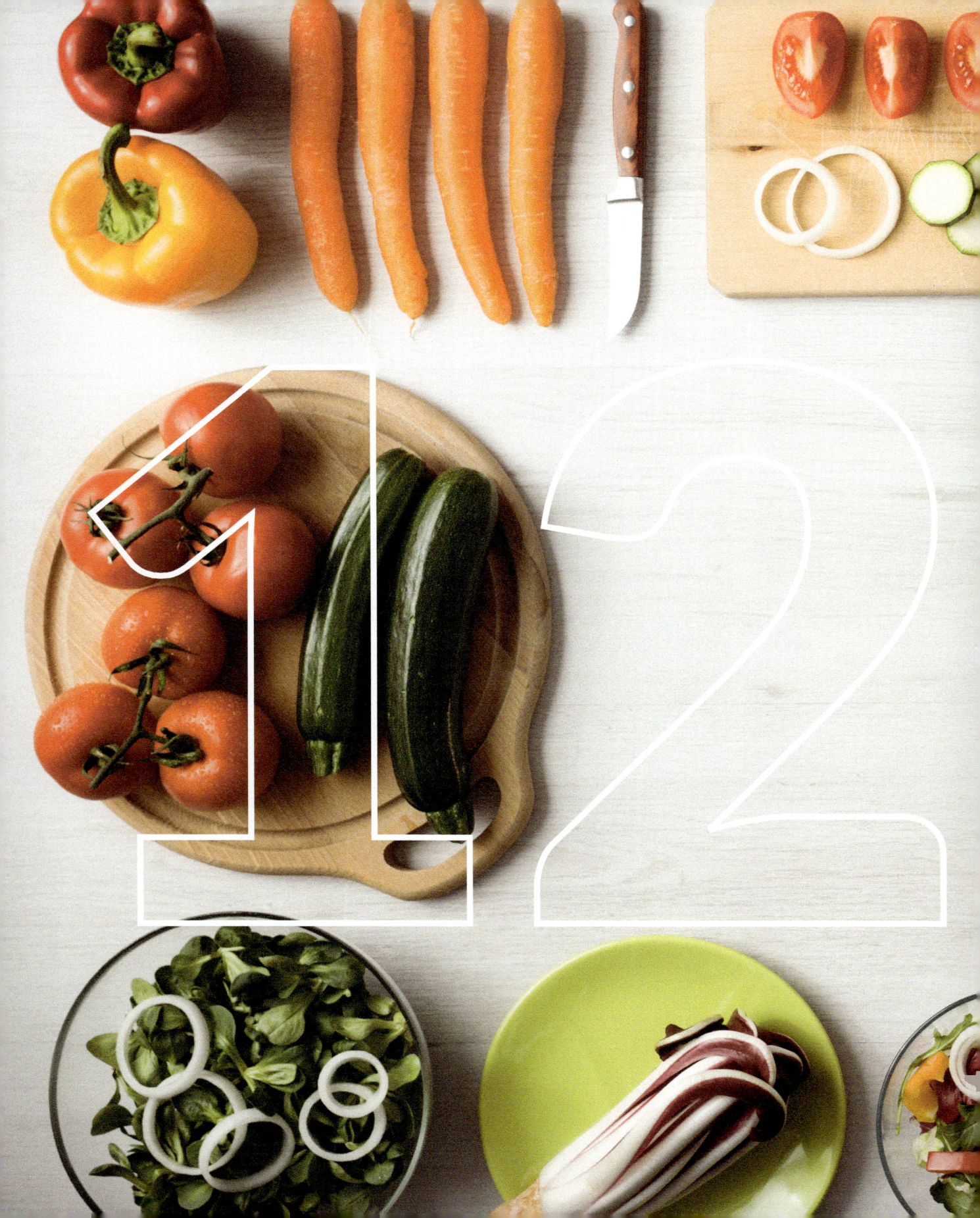

CHAPTER TWELVE

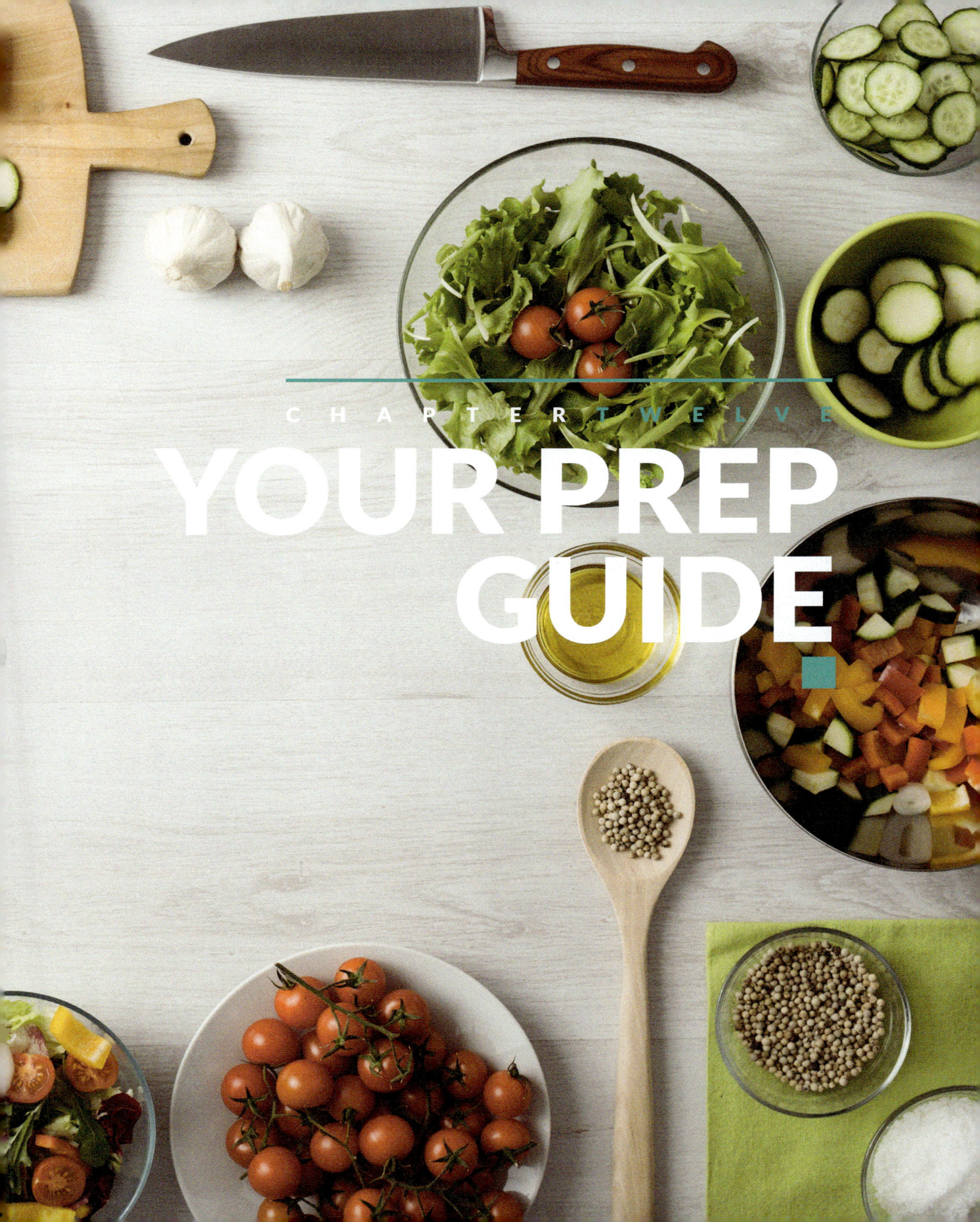

YOUR PREP GUIDE

12.1
GET PREPPED

Being prepared does not mean that you need the 12 Tupperware boxes of chicken and broccoli seen frequently on social media. It simply means thinking ahead and planning, so you don't get caught off guard. Being prepared means that when the unpredictable happens, you can deal with it.

Step 1 - Plan your week

Take one hour from, let's say Sunday, and sit down to arrange meal ideas and review numbers for the following week. You need to look at your schedule and plan accordingly using something like the meal planner provided in the resource section. Are you going to be busy and home late? Are you going to be travelling on the days you are going to the gym? Are you competing away? From this you can decide which days you need to plan for.

Step 2 - Plan your meals

Once you have an idea of how your week is going to look, plan your meals around your schedule. You don't need to calculate the kcals and macros for each day or meal, but have a rough idea about what you need to prepare.

We recommend a list of "go-to" meals for breakfasts, lunches and evening meals that are well balanced and include each of the main food groups, lean protein, high fibre carbohydrates, fruit, vegetables and a small amount of fat. These should be meals that you know well, are easy to prepare and will stop the *'what can I have!'* moments.

Weekly Planner

Meal	Monday	Tuesday	Wednesday	Thursday	Friday	Saturday	Sunday
1							
2							
3							
4							
5							
6							
Macros							

These don't have to be Michelin star standard, just simple tasty dishes.

Breakfast options
- Breakfast smoothie
- Oats, whey protein, milk and handful of berries'
- Eggs on toast with wilted spinach and mushrooms
- Fruit and yoghurt parfait

Lunch options
- Lean meat (chicken/turkey) sandwiches or wraps with a piece of fruit
- Protein packed salads – Spinach and rocket base, cherry tomatoes, red onion and peppers, lean meat or fish, balsamic vinegar/olive oil and lemon juice. The combinations are endless.
- Leftovers from the evening before

Evening meal
- *Grilled chicken with sweet potato mash and mixed greens*
- *Herb crusted white fish with new potatoes and roasted veg*
- *Bolognese with spiralised veg and parmesan*

Snacks
- *Greek yoghurt and nuts*
- *Boiled eggs and a piece of fruit*
- *Jerky or biltong and a piece of fruit*
- *Vegetable sticks and hummus or homemade tzatziki*

Good nutrition doesn't necessarily have to be complicated, instead it should be something you are likely to stick with. If it does become boring or tiresome then add one more "go to" meal to your list. Over time you'll be able to develop a whole list of different meals. If you do struggle with ideas or creativity then use resources like Yummly, Pinterest and BuzzFeed for some inspiration.

Top tip - Start adding your recipes to an Excel spreadsheet along with a list of ingredients to help writing your shopping list.

Step 3 - Prep your meals

It's a good idea to organise at least part of your week with a shopping list. By doing this you know what you need to buy. Your next task is to take a trip to the supermarket using the shopping list you have made. Online shopping is a great option that enables you to save your shopping list, so you can reorder the same foods each week without the hassle of even visiting the shops.

Batch Preparation

Batch preparation is a simple and effective strategy to make things easy for the week ahead. Good examples include:

One pot dishes - Make one big dish such as chilli con carne, Bolognese, curry or stew and then portion it up before freezing it. It's as simple as removing a meal you fancy from the freezer the night before and letting it defrost safely in the fridge before heating it up.

Chicken breasts - Place chicken breasts on a baking tray, drizzle with olive oil, add salt and pepper or any spice or herb mix. Bake for 20-30 minutes at 180c.

Potatoes - Chop, drizzle with olive oil, add salt and bake at 180c for around 45 minutes. Or boil until soft and add butter.

Roasted vegetables – Chop a selection of vegetables and lay out on a baking tray. Drizzle with olive oil and play with herb mixes to suit your taste. Bake for 20-30 minutes at 180c.

Vegetable Accompaniments - Fill Tupperware boxes with chopped vegetables and store them in the fridge. It's as simple as grabbing a handful each day to add to your lunch box for snacks or lunches. Alternatively, you could buy frozen vegetables which are just as healthy (and stay fresh for longer). Simply add a few handfuls to your chosen protein source each day.

Hard boiled eggs – Hard boils are one of the easiest and most nutritious snacks on the go. Simply boil 5-10 and store in the fridge ready to take to work each day.

Top tip – Adding baking soda to the water makes peeling the eggs effortless.

Building Your Box Nutrition kitchen

Make your preparation a lot easier with this list of kitchen appliances.

Kitchen scales – A set of digital food scales makes tracking your food intake a lot easier and is a great tool to help you understand food portions.

A set of measuring spoons and cups – If you don't have any of these you could use an old protein powder scoop or invest in a set (they shouldn't be expensive). Measuring cups or spoons are useful when working out portion sizes, by using these you will know how many scoops of rice or pasta for example, you should be adding to your meals.

Smoothie maker – These are worth the investment. Something you will use time and again, smoothie makers are superb for quick, easy snacks, nutrient rich shakes, fruit smoothies, even breakfast porridge and more.

Plastic Tupperware/containers – Get ready to meet your new best friend in the kitchen! We suggest you buy a set of different size Tupperware if you don't already have some. Tupperware is an excellent way of keeping food fresh, neatly contained and means you can easily transport food for when you're not at home; use these for lunch, snacks and for storing food you want to eat later.

Protein shaker – If you don't have one of these, use a plastic bottle (it works just as well) but keep it really clean after each shake as residue can build up.

Soup maker – A great tool for ensuring you get enough vegetables in your diet. Sauté an onion, stick of celery and a carrot, add stock, a selection of other vegetables and leave for twenty minutes. It's that simple. Perfect when you have leftovers at the end of week.

To help you with your planning for the week, we have included a shopping list and meal planner in the resource section. It is not exhaustive but gives you a good starting point for each food group.

To sum up

1. Choose which days you need to prepare for in advance and make note of it in your meal planner.

2. Are you going to the gym? What do you need to prepare?

3. Are you going to be late any times this week? What can you prepare?

4. Are you going away at all this week? What do you need to prepare?

5. Record what meals you want to have this week in your meal planner. Use the sample meal plan and websites like Pinterest and BBC Good Food for recipe ideas.

6. Using your shopping list as a guide, buy your ingredients for the week.

CHAPTER THIRTEEN

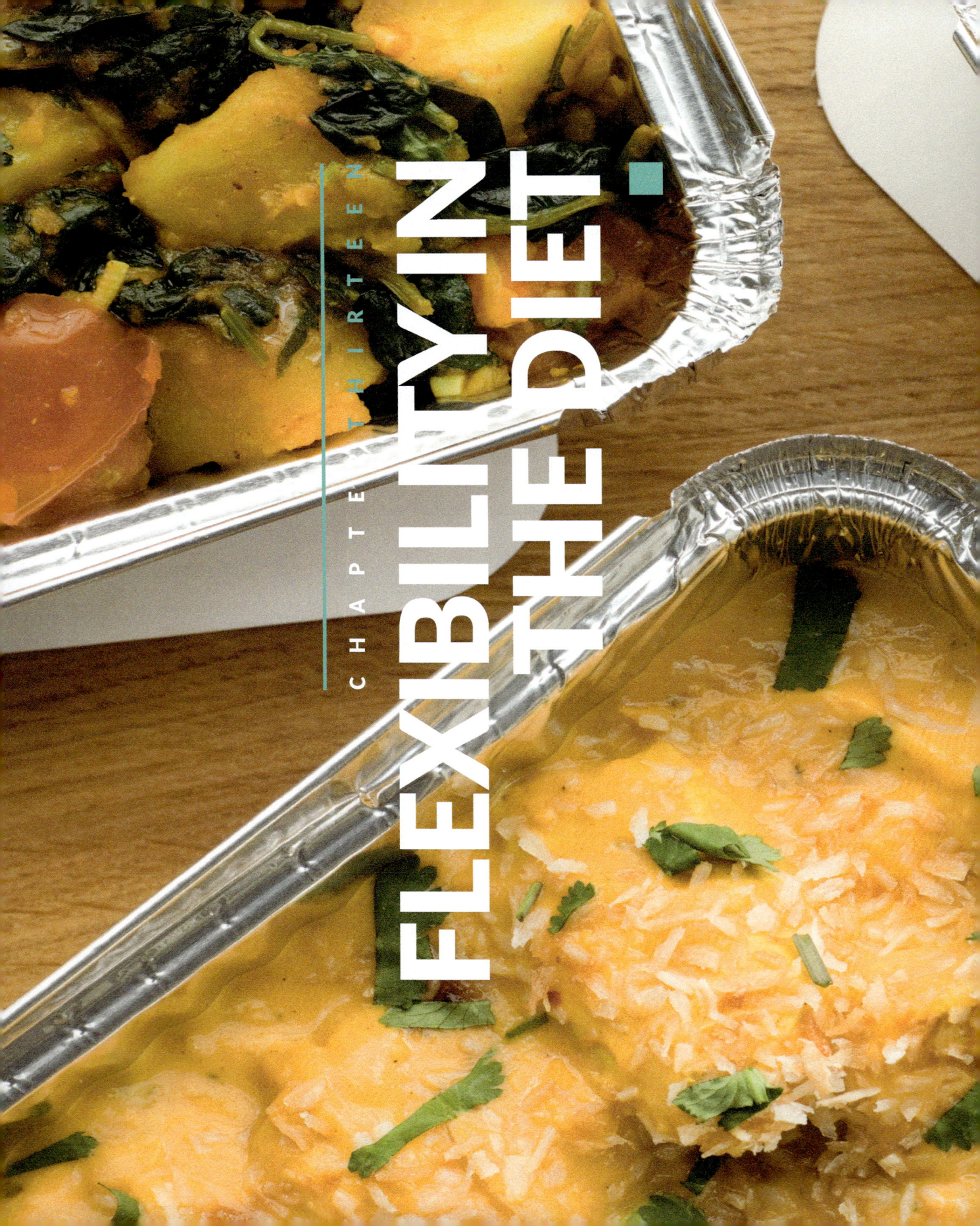

FLEXIBILITY IN THE DIET

13

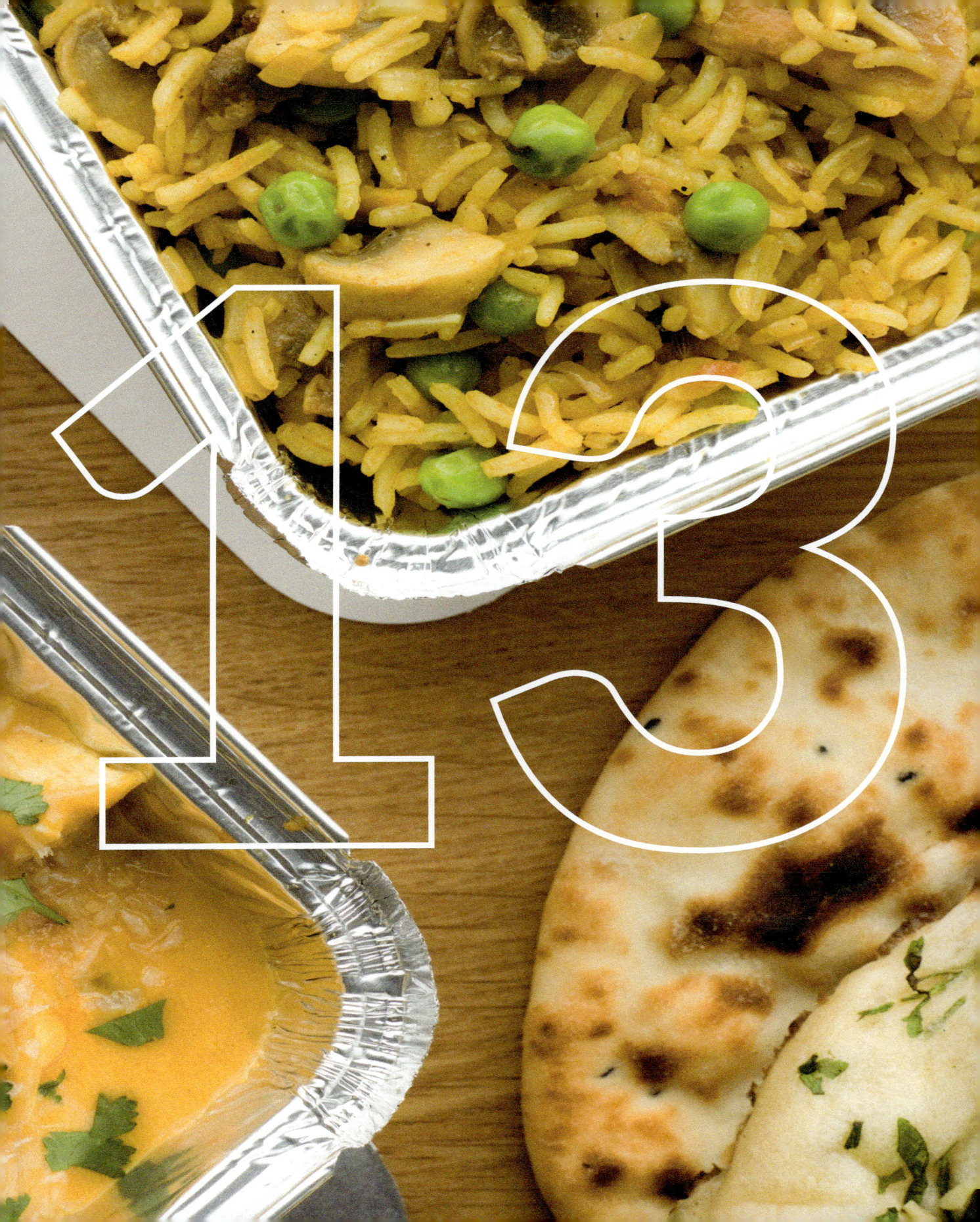

13.1
THE BALANCED APPROACH

At Box, we strongly support a balanced approach to eating, with no food being banned. However, you can't always have your cake and eat it, sometimes literally.

Flexibility in your diet without sabotaging results

Unfortunately, the likelihood of being able to sport a six-pack or bikini body whilst overindulging on Pop Tarts and Oreo's is pretty low. However, that's not to say you can't have a bit of both.

But how?

1. Find your cost of getting into shape

What are you willing to sacrifice to get the results you want? We don't always know immediately what it takes to get in shape. This can create a false impression of the effort required which can affect our motivation going forward.

Try and identify what it will take to reach your goals. Obviously losing a few pounds and feeling healthier requires less time and dedication than a chiselled set of abs and a 2 x your bodyweight squat, but knowing your cost of getting in shape will also make you more at ease with what you need to do.

Precision Nutrition have created a fantastic infographic helping to show what it takes to get to certain levels of body fat: **https://www.precisionnutrition.com/cost-of-getting-lean-infographic**

2. Don't ban foods
There is no such thing as a bad food, just bad habits. Saying you will never eat this or that food again (pizza, crisps, ice cream, peanut butter) will only make you to want those foods even more. And guess what happens when you crack… A spoon and an empty tub of Ben and Jerry's.

3. Don't strive for perfection
Imperfection is completely normal and should be accepted. Slow "imperfect" progress is far better than striving for perfection which will inevitably fail and leave you unstuck. Don't view your diet as black or white where a bad day means all is lost. Just because you have had a packet of biscuits it does not mean you have to wait until Monday to restart your diet. If you have a bad day, simply accept it and move on.

4. Drop the quick fix mentality
The choices we make over months, not one day or one hour, dictate the way our bodies will look and feel. Looking for diet pills, crash diets and jumping straight into an excessive exercise regime inevitably leads to failure. A drastic drop in kcals is not sustainable and will more than likely lead to subsequent weight gain or a performance decrement. Don't let quick fix thinking distract you from the hard work of changing unhealthy behaviours, which are the root cause of weight gain and poor performance.

5. Substitute

Look to substitute hyper-palatable foods (cakes, biscuits, crisps, chocolate) for lower kcal snacks and drinks. Although these may not all be deemed healthy, it's better to have the odd one of these than to consistently overeat.

- Sweet snacks under 100 kcals – popcorn, low kcal bags of crisps, snack jacks, 10 kcal jelly pots, frozen grapes
- Make your own crisps by baking thinly sliced vegetables or fruit
- Look for high protein low kcal snacks – biltong, Greek yoghurt/quark/skyr, boiled eggs
- Use zero kcal sweeteners, syrups and flavour drops to help give some extra flavour to your food without using up too many kcals
- Opt for zero kcal drinks – Look for diet varieties if you are out or just craving a sweet drink

6. Get by

Sometimes you just need something to get by until there is something better available. How many times have you eaten your afternoon snack too early or forgotten to prepare it all together? Your options are limited and mostly unhealthy. In these situations, a few strategies that can help are:

1. Drink tea or coffee
2. Chew gum
3. Brush your teeth
4. Drink water
5. Suck it up

7. Checks and balances

Learn to be more flexible with your eating. Being restrictive in certain areas enables you to be more flexible in others.

For example:
- Remove carbohydrates from your evening meal so you can have dessert
- Eat the burger without the bread so you can have dessert
- Having no afternoon snack so you can have a bedtime snack
- Don't have carbohydrates at lunch so you can increase them in the evening
- Skip carbs at breakfast so you can have a few drinks at night

8. Be strict with being balanced

This may seem like an oxymoron, but an "if it fits your macros (IIFYM)" approach can allow you to fit in some of the "bad foods" you like without deviating too far from your macronutrient goals for the day. What this means is that providing you stay within your macros, you can eat whichever foods you like (within reason!).

9. Get strict for 8-12 weeks

Set a goal for yourself, give yourself a time frame and give it everything. It's not forever!

10. Build an environment conducive with your goals

Do you have access to sweet treats? Are they in your house? Usually if something is in reach and doesn't take much effort to grab, you will eat it (and keep eating it). So don't buy it. The harder it is to get hold of a food the less likely it is you will eat it.

11. Drink wisely

Alcohol inhibits protein and glycogen synthesis affecting recovery and the building of new muscle, especially after resistance training (21, 22). However, the odd night out is not going to have a huge effect on your progress. If body composition or weight loss is the goal, then maintaining a kcal deficit is key. Therefore, if you plan to drink make a conscious effort to reduce calorific foods the day before, of and after drinking, while also choosing lower kcal drinks where possible.

Kcal balancing

Kcal balance over one week is more important than day-to-day management. Overeating for one day will have a negligible impact on your results compared to consistently overeating over the week. To help you manage this, you can adjust your daily targets while still reaching the same weekly average. This is a good strategy if you plan on going out or if you feel you need to compensate for a day of overeating. We recommend not to drop kcals more than 20% of your daily target.

Example

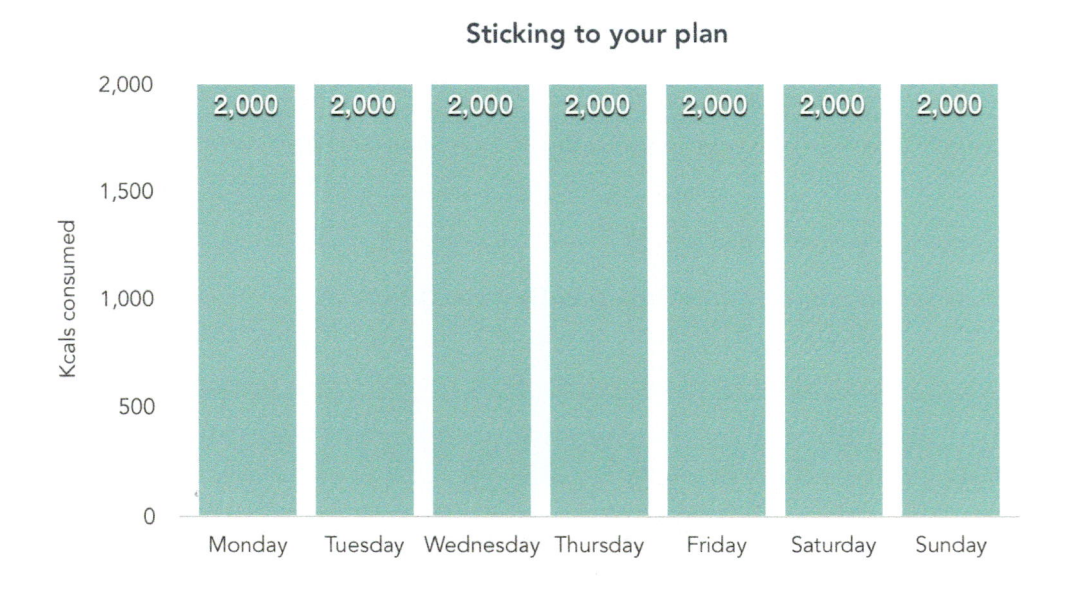

Sticking to your plan

Day	Kcals consumed
Monday	2,000
Tuesday	2,000
Wednesday	2,000
Thursday	2,000
Friday	2,000
Saturday	2,000
Sunday	2,000

Planning for the weekend

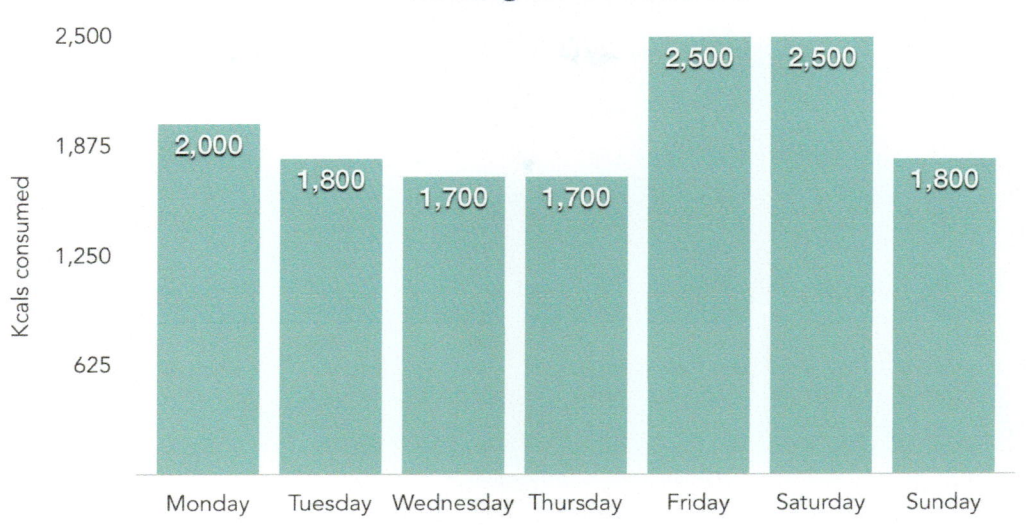

Day	Kcals consumed
Monday	2,000
Tuesday	1,800
Wednesday	1,700
Thursday	1,700
Friday	2,500
Saturday	2,500
Sunday	1,800

Correcting for overeating

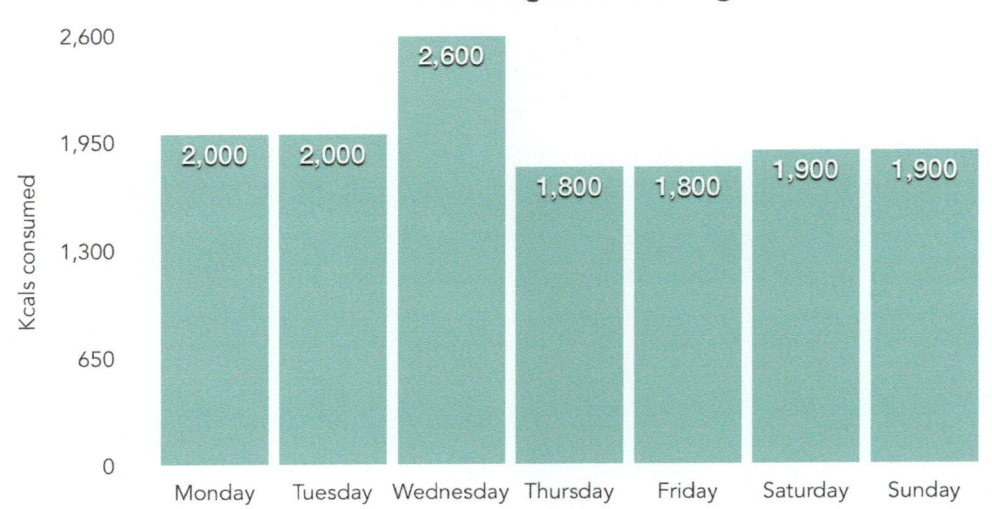

Day	Kcals consumed
Monday	2,000
Tuesday	2,000
Wednesday	2,600
Thursday	1,800
Friday	1,800
Saturday	1,900
Sunday	1,900

flexibility in the diet

14

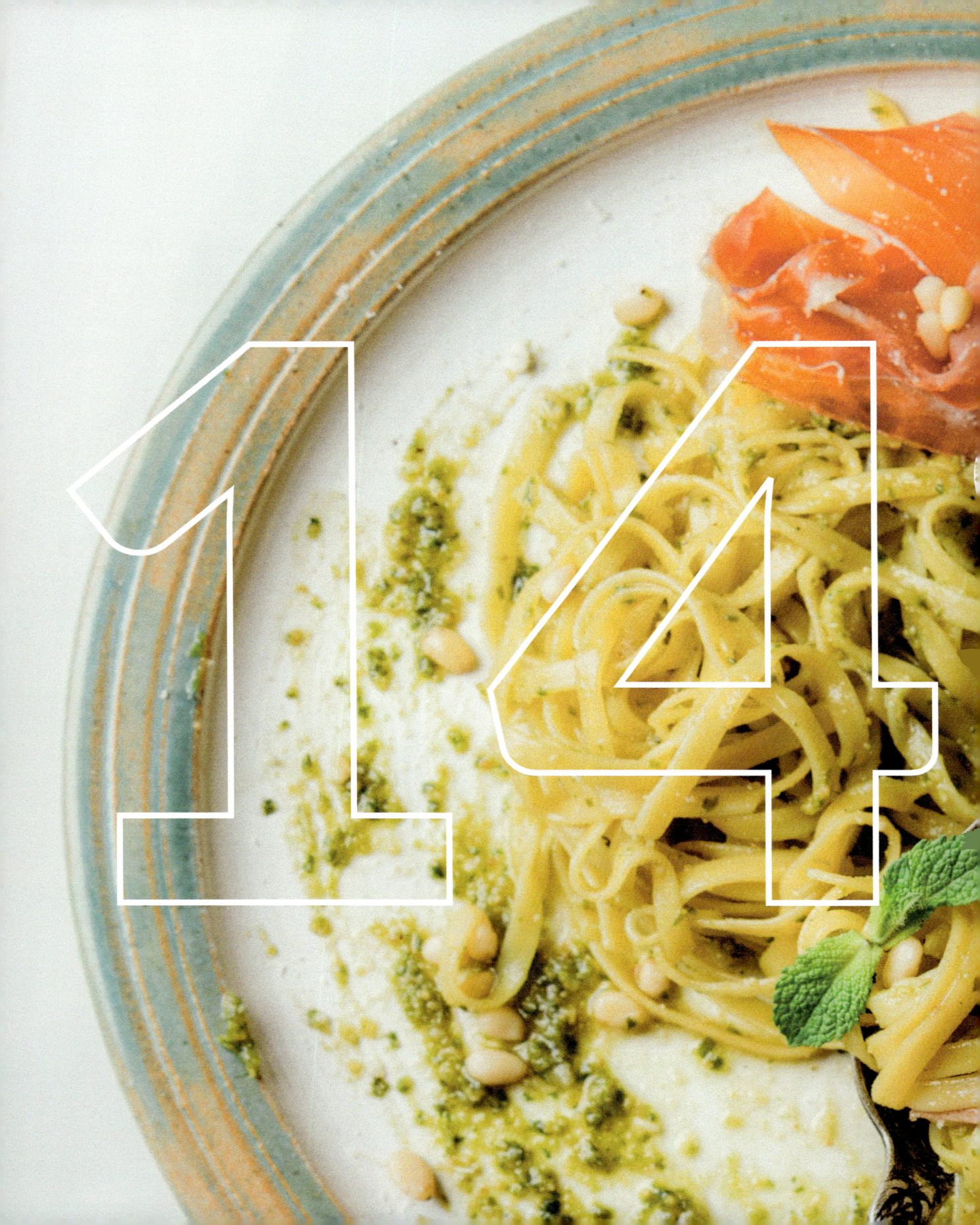

CHAPTER FOURTEEN
EATING OUT

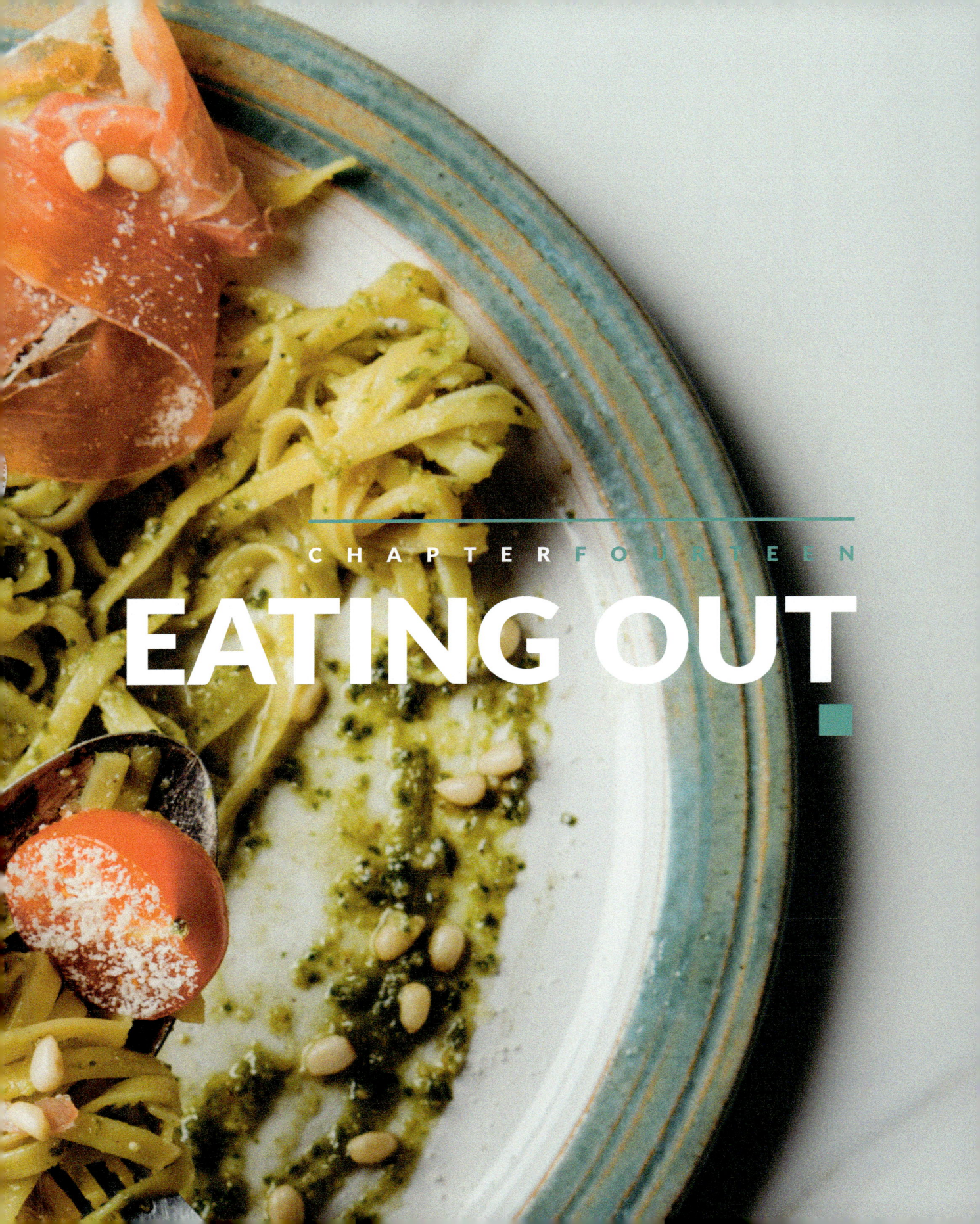

14.1
EATING ON THE GO

When your daily routine is similar it can be quite easy to stick to your meal plan. However, it's inevitable that life will get in the way. Work lunches, drinks, cakes in the office, birthday brunches and meals out with your other half can make it difficult to stick to your plan. So it's good to have some strategies in place to help avoid sabotaging your results.

Strategies for eating on the road

1. Eat a balanced meal before you leave the house
If you're not hungry when you go out, you're less likely to overeat, which is why it is a good idea to have a balanced meal before leaving the house. When building your meal, think about balancing your meals that include the main food groups: one protein portion, one fat portion, one carbohydrate portion and a portion of vegetables where possible.

Take snacks with you:
- *Boiled eggs*
- *Protein shake or bar*
- *Carrots and hummus*
- *Vegetable sticks*
- *Nuts and seeds*
- *Biltong or nitrate free meat slices*

- *Chicken breasts cut into chunks*
- *Tins of tuna/mackerel*
- *Fruit*
- *Low fat Greek yoghurt*
- *Cottage cheese*
- *Buy a cool bag if you're going to be out for a while*

Simple lunches on the go

Make your own green salad
- *Green base – leafy greens/lettuce/spinach/rocket/watercress*
- *Optional added vegetables – tomatoes/cucumber/peppers/red onion/spring onion /beetroot/carrots*
- *Protein portion – chicken, turkey, steak slices, tofu, tuna, salmon, low fat cottage cheese*
- *Fat portion – sprinkle of seeds/nuts/olives/cheese/half an avocado/pesto*
- *Carbohydrate portion – new potatoes, sweet potatoes, chickpeas, couscous, butternut squash, rice*

Make a sandwich
- *Carbohydrate portion – 2-4 slices of wholemeal bread*
- *Protein portion – chicken, steak slices, ham, tofu, tuna, salmon*
- *Fat portion – cheese, half an avocado, butter, mayonnaise*
- *Green option – lettuce/spinach/rocket/watercress*
- *Added vegetables – tomatoes/cucumber/peppers/red onion/spring onion/radishes/beetroot/carrots*
- *Optional added fruit*

Strategies for when buying your lunch from a shop

If you haven't prepped, ask yourself what's best, better and worst? What's the best option that is available to you in this current situation? This doesn't have to be perfect. Try and look for supermarkets, then mini supermarkets as petrol stations and local newsagents are unlikely to have a good selection.

Remember the steps in your meal plan
1. Protein portion
2. Fat portion
3. Carbohydrate portion
4. Vegetable portion
5. Optional fruit portion

Checking food labels

A simple task like reading a food label enables you to make more informed choices about what you eat and drink. Typically, the front of a food label will contain the number of kcals, saturated fat, sugar, salt and the % of your reference Intake / Recommended Daily Amount (RDA).

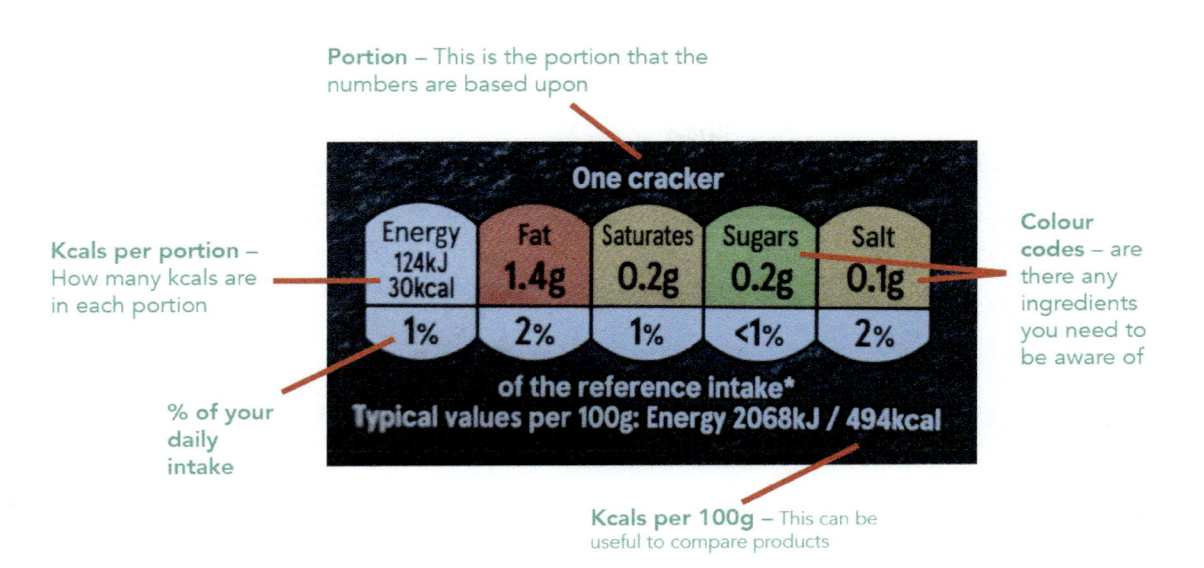

Portion – This is the portion that the numbers are based upon

Kcals per portion – How many kcals are in each portion

Colour codes – are there any ingredients you need to be aware of

% of your daily intake

Kcals per 100g – This can be useful to compare products

The colour-coded nutritional information tells you at a glance if the food has high, medium or low amounts of the nutrients mentioned above:

- *Red means high amounts*
- *Amber means moderate amounts*
- *Green means low amounts*

What is high and low

	Low	Moderate	High
Fat	3g or less	3.1-17.5g	>17.5g
Saturated Fat	1.5g or less	1.6-5g	>5g
Sugar	5g or less	5.1-22.5g	>22.5g
Salt	0.3g or less	0.3-1.5g	>1.5g

For healthier options, typically choose products with more greens and fewer reds. A red label does not necessarily mean that you cannot have this food, you just need to recognise that it is high in a certain nutrient. This may mean you have to reduce the amount of this type of food later in the day. For example, if you have a food that is high in fat, you may need to opt for lower fat foods later in the day.

You must also be aware that some foods like cheese, oily fish or meat may be high in fat but are also high in protein and other essential nutrients.

Check the back

The nutrition label on the back or side of the food will contain the ingredients list, nutrients per 100g, per serving/portion and number of portions per pack. Use this label to check the protein content of the food and help make comparisons with other foods.

Going out for dinner checklist

Socialising can easily derail your dietary adherence, however there are several things you can do to limit the damage, still enjoy yourself and avoid any guilt.

1. Don't worry

One meal doesn't ruin your progress, just like one salad doesn't make you healthy. What you do consistently is what counts. If you're having the odd meal out, then try not let it bother you and just enjoy these occasions.

2. Daily vs weekly calories

It's your weekly caloric intake that matters, not your daily count. If you overeat for one day it will have a negligible effect. To help with this, use the kcal balancing strategy mentioned in the previous chapter and create a buffer leading up to this day. Dropping your kcals by 200-250 for a few days beforehand gives you more flexibility for your night out.

3. Check the menu
Do your research and check the menu before you go out for dinner, so you have a better idea about what to choose beforehand.

4. Avoid combination foods
Try and avoid meals that are high in both fat and carbohydrates. These hyper-palatable, high kcal foods are the major culprits responsible for fat gain. These include most desserts, pies, pastries, chips and fried food.

5. Choose a leaner source of protein
Always go for leaner cuts of meat and fish like chicken, turkey, fish or seafood to help curb additional kcals.

6. Make the swap
If you're worried about excess kcals, swap a portion of starchy carbohydrates or chips for green vegetables. Also look to substitute full sugar drinks for zero or lower kcal alternatives.

7. Be mindful of condiments
As previously mentioned, condiments and dressings can quickly add up in kcals meaning you should operate with caution when adding them to your food.

CHAPTER FIFTEEN

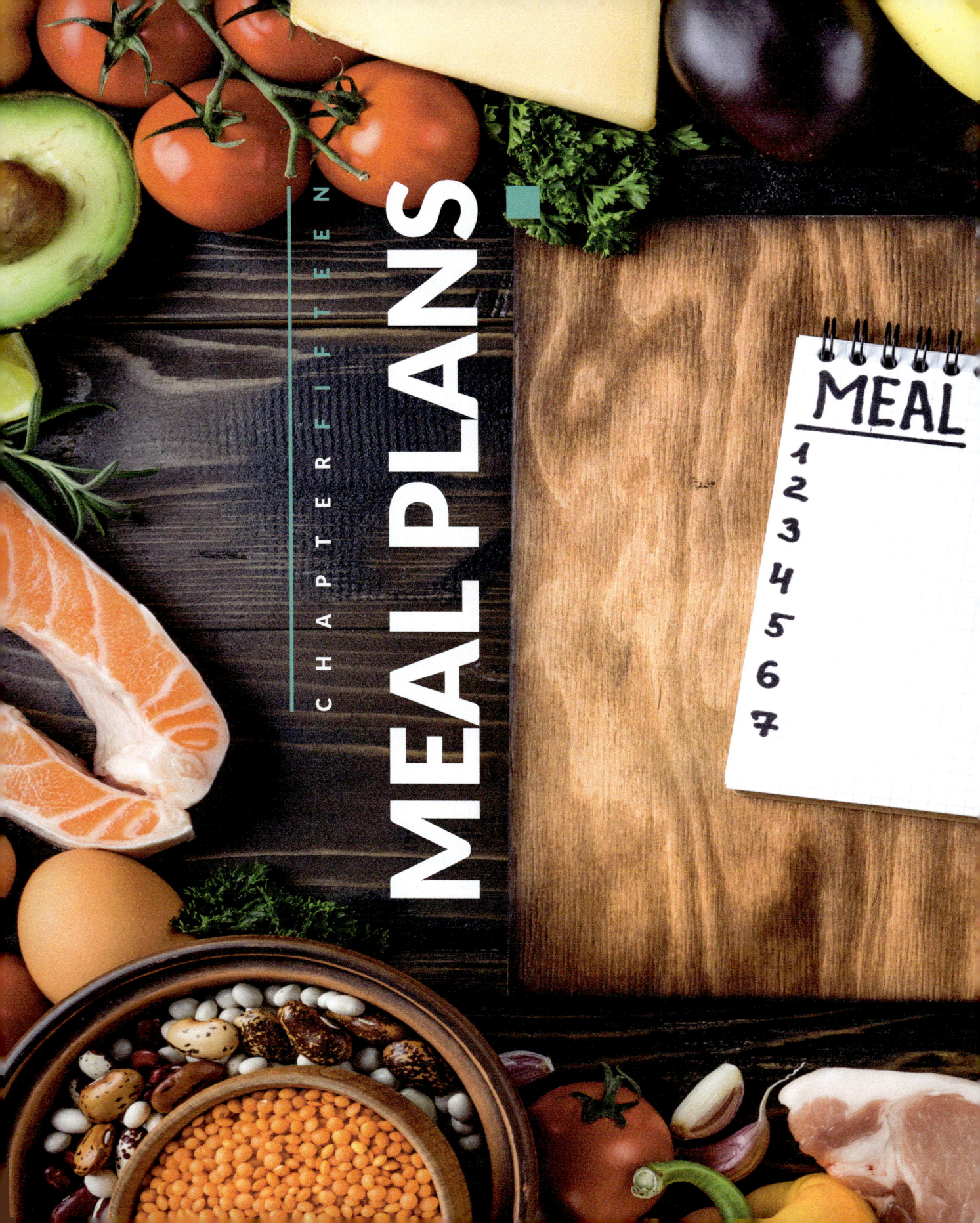

MEAL PLANS

15

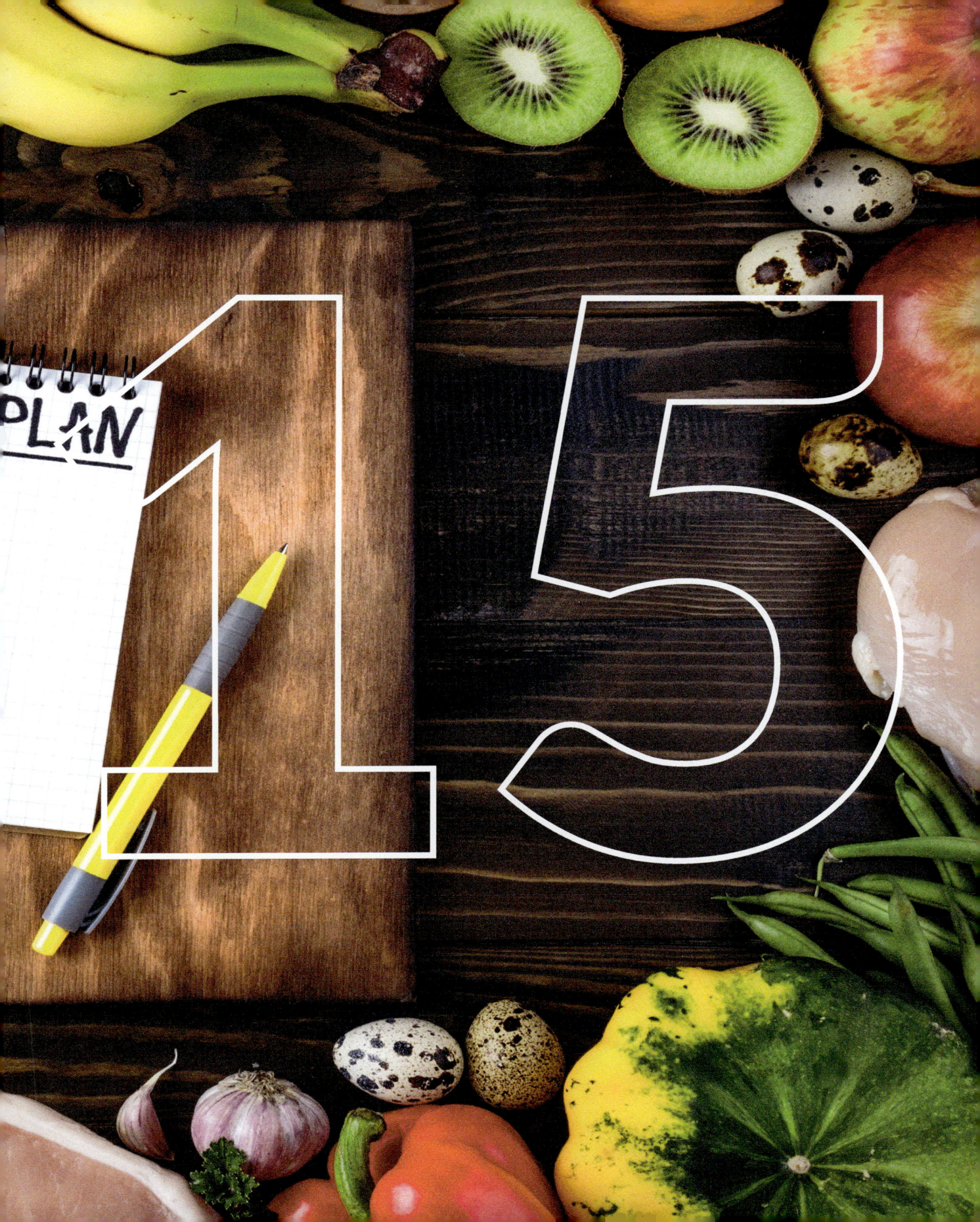

1,500 kcal plan

Food Name	Grams	Measure	Kcals	Carbs	Protein	Fat
Breakfast - Egg frittata						
Eggs chicken white raw	64	2x average egg	28	0	7	0
Eggs chicken whole raw	114	2x average size 3	150	0	14	10
Peas frozen boiled in unsalted water	25	1x tablespoon	18	3	1	0
Spinach baby raw	20	1x cup	3	0	1	0
		Meal Total	**198kcal**	**2.7g**	**23.2g**	**10.6g**
Lunch - Tuna couscous salad						
Cheese Feta	30	1x 5 1cm cubes	75	0	5	6
Couscous plain raw	60	0.7x average portion	213	43	7	1
Cucumber raw flesh and skin	55	1x 1/2 cup slices	8	1	1	0
Lemon juice fresh	15	1x tablespoon	1	0	0	0
Peppers capsicum red raw	24	2x ring slice	5	1	0	0
Rocket leaves raw	20	1x cup	4	0	1	0
Tomatoes cherry raw	75	5x cherry tomato	18	3	1	0
Tuna canned in brine drained	72	1x small can (100g) drained	78	0	18	1
		Meal Total	**397kcal**	**37.4g**	**36.9g**	**11.1g**
Afternoon snack - Rice cakes with peanut butter						
Blueberries	50	4.8x 15 blueberries	21	5	0	0
Peanut butter wholegrain	20	1x tablespoon	121	1	5	11
Rice cakes plain low salt	18	1x average Portion	63	13	1	1
		Meal Total	**205kcal**	**19g**	**6.8g**	**11.3g**
Evening meal - Turkey chilli and basmati rice						
Cajun spice mix	8.1	1x tablespoon	17	2	1	0
Onions red raw	18.8	2x sandwich filling	7	1	0	0
Peppers bell raw mixed	30	2.5x ring slice	8	1	0	0
Rice white basmati raw	65	1x serving	222	49	5	0
Tomatoes canned whole contents	95	1x average Portion	20	4	1	0
Turkey mince raw 7% fat	200	0.5x medium Pack	309	0	46	14
		Meal Total	**581kcal**	**58g**	**53g**	**15g**
Bed time treat						
Ice cream dairy vanilla soft scoop	75	1x average serving	129	16	2	6
		Meal Total	**129kcal**	**15.9g**	**2.4g**	**6.2g**
		Plan total	**1515kcal**	**144g**	**118g**	**52g**

2,000 kcal plan

Food Name	Grams	Measure	Kcals	Carbs	Protein	Fat
Breakfast - Overnight oats and chia pudding						
Chia seeds	10	1x tablespoon	39	1	2	3
Mangoes ripe raw flesh only	52	1x average Portion	31	7	0	0
Milk semi-skimmed pasteurised average	135	1x on cereal (30-35g portion)	64	6	5	2
Oat flakes rolled	60	1x 3/4 cup	224	39	7	5
Yogurt Greek plain 0% fat	45	1x tablespoon	26	2	5	0
		Meal Total	384kcal	54g	18.2g	10.4g
Lunch - Chicken noodle salad						
Carrots old raw	67	1x medium carrot	24	5	0	0
Chicken breast grilled without skin meat only	90	1x small fillet	122	0	27	2
Courgette raw	80	1x medium portion / NHS Serving	14	1	1	0
Lemon juice fresh	5	1x teaspoon	0	0	0	0
Noodles egg medium dried boiled in unsalted water	100	0.4x average serving	162	33	6	1
Peanut butter wholegrain	15	1x heaped teaspoon	91	1	4	8
Soy sauce light and dark varieties	6	1x average Portion	5	1	0	0
Spring onions bulbs and tops raw	10	1x average	3	0	0	0
Sweet chilli sauce	7	1x teaspoon	17	4	0	0
		Meal Total	438kcal	45g	38.4g	11.4g
Snack - vegetable sticks and hummus						
Carrots old raw	120	1x large carrot	43	9	1	0
Cucumber raw flesh and skin	100	1.8x 1/2 cup slices	14	1	1	1
Hummus retail	60	2x tablespoon	178	5	5	16
		Meal total	234kcal	14.9g	6.3g	16.6g
Turkey burger						
Bread rolls wholemeal	80	1x large petit pain	192	34	8	3
Cheese Halloumi	30	0.4x 1/2cup	94	0	7	7

Food Name	Grams	Measure	Kcals	Carbs	Protein	Fat
Courgette raw	20	2x per slice	4	0	0	0
Mushrooms white raw	16	1x average	1	0	0	0
Onions raw	15	1x slice or in sandwich/wrap	6	1	0	0
Tomato ketchup	8	1x teaspoon	10	2	0	0
Turkey mince raw 4% fat	100	0.3x Medium Pack	130	0	24	4
		Meal Total	**436kcal**	**38g**	**39.9g**	**13.8g**
Workout snack - Rice cakes and whey protein shake						
Milk semi-skimmed pasteurised average	200		95	9	7	3
Rice cake Bunalun Dark Chocolate	66	4x rice cake	310	37	4	16
Whey protein isolate powder	30	1x average serving/scoop	114	0	27	0
		Meal Total	**235kcal**	**28.3g**	**3.2g**	**12.1g**
		Plan total	**2010kcal**	**199g**	**141g**	**72g**

2,500 kcal plan

Food Name	Grams	Measure	Kcals	Carbs	Protein	Fat
Breakfast - Overnight oats and chia pudding						
Overnight oats						
Chia seeds	20	2x tablespoon	78	2	4	6
Mangoes ripe raw flesh only	52	1x average Portion	31	7	0	0
Milk semi-skimmed pasteurised average	180	6x In tea/coffee	85	8	6	3
Oat flakes rolled	80	1x cup	299	51	9	7
Yogurt greek plain 0% fat	45	1x tablespoon	26	2	5	0
		Meal Total	**518kcal**	**70g**	**23.8g**	**15.9g**
Snack - vegetable sticks and hummus						
Carrots old raw	120	1x large carrot	43	9	1	0
Cucumber raw flesh and skin	100	1.8x 1/2 cup slices	14	1	1	1
Hummus retail	60	2x tablespoon	178	5	5	16
		Meal Total	**234kcal**	**14.9g**	**6.3g**	**16.6g**
Lunch - Chicken noodle salad						

Food Name	Grams	Measure	Kcals	Carbs	Protein	Fat
Carrots old raw	67	1x NHS serving (1 medium carrot)	24	5	0	0
Chicken breast grilled without skin meat only	120	1x medium fillet	162	0	35	2
Courgette raw	80	1x medium portion / NHS serving	14	1	1	0
Lemon juice fresh	5	1x teaspoon	0	0	0	0
Noodles egg medium dried boiled in unsalted water	140	0.5x average serving	227	46	8	1
Peanut butter wholegrain	15	1x heaped teaspoon	91	1	4	8
Soy sauce light and dark varieties	6	1x average portion	5	1	0	0
Spring onions bulbs and tops raw	10	1x average	3	0	0	0
Sweet chilli sauce	7	1x teaspoon	17	4	0	0
		Meal Total	**543kcal**	**58g**	**50g**	**12.4g**
Evening meal - Turkey burger						
Bread rolls wholemeal	160	2x large petit pain	384	67	17	5
Cheese Halloumi	30	0.4x 1/2cup	94	0	7	7
Courgette raw	20	2x per slice	4	0	0	0
Mushrooms white raw	32	2x average	2	0	0	0
Onions raw	30	2x slice or in sandwich/wrap	11	2	0	0
Tomato ketchup	16	2x teaspoon	19	4	0	0
Turkey mince raw 4% fat	150	0.6x small pack	195	0	35	6
		Meal Total	**709kcal**	**75g**	**60g**	**18.5g**
Workout snack - Pre or post workout						
Milk semi-skimmed pasteurised average	200		95	9	7	3
Rice cake Bunalun Dark Chocolate	66	4x rice cake	310	37	4	16
Whey protein isolate powder	30	1x average serving/scoop	114	0	27	0
		Meal Total	**518kcal**	**47g**	**38.2g**	**19.8g**
		Plan total	**2523kcal**	**265g**	**178g**	**83g**

3000 kcal plan

Food Name	Grams	Measure	Kcals	Carbs	Protein	Fat
Breakfast - Overnight oats and chia pudding						
Chia seeds	20	2x tablespoon	78	2	4	6
Mangoes ripe raw flesh only	52	1x average portion	31	7	0	0
Milk semi-skimmed pasteurised average	180	6x In tea/coffee	85	8	6	3
Oat flakes rolled	80	1x cup	299	51	9	7
Yogurt greek plain 0% fat	45	1x tablespoon	26	2	5	0
		Meal Total	518kcal	70g	23.8g	15.9g
Snack - vegetable sticks and hummus						
Carrots old raw	120	1x large carrot	43	9	1	0
Cream crackers	21	3x cracker	92	13	2	3
Cucumber raw flesh and skin	100	1.8x 1/2 cup slices	14	1	1	1
Hummus retail	60	2x tablespoon	178	5	5	16
		Meal Total	326kcal	28.3g	8.1g	20.1g
Lunch - Chicken noodle salad						
Carrots old raw	67	1x NHS serving (1 medium carrot)	24	5	0	0
Chicken breast grilled without skin meat only	120	1x medium fillet	162	0	35	2
Courgette raw	80	1x medium portion / NHS Serving	14	1	1	0
Lemon juice fresh	5	1x teaspoon	0	0	0	0
Noodles egg medium dried boiled in unsalted water	180	0.6x average serving	292	59	10	2
Peanut butter wholegrain	15	1x heaped teaspoon	91	1	4	8
Soy sauce light and dark varieties	6	1x average portion	5	1	0	0
Spring onions bulbs and tops raw	10	1x average	3	0	0	0
Sweet chilli sauce	7	1x teaspoon	17	4	0	0
		Meal Total	608kcal	71g	52g	12.8g
Evening meal - Turkey burger						
Bread rolls wholemeal	160	2x large petit pain	384	67	17	5
Courgette raw	20	2x per slice	4	0	0	0
Mushrooms white raw	32	2x average	2	0	0	0
Onions raw	30	2x slice or in sandwich/wrap	11	2	0	0
Tomato ketchup	16	2x teaspoon	19	4	0	0
Turkey mince raw 4% fat	150	0.6x Small pack	195	0	35	6
		Meal Total	614kcal	75g	53g	11.4g

Food Name	Grams	Measure	Kcals	Carbs	Protein	Fat
Workout snack - Rice cakes						
Rice cake Belgian Dark Chocolate	66	4x rice cake	310	37	4	16
		Meal Total	**310kcal**	**37.4g**	**4.2g**	**16g**
Post workout shake						
Bananas flesh only	200	2x Medium	171	40	2	0
Milk semi-skimmed pasteurised average	200		95	9	7	3
Whey protein isolate powder	30	1x average	114	0	27	0
		Meal Total	**380kcal**	**49g**	**36.4g**	**4.1g**
Bed time treat						
Ice cream dairy vanilla soft scoop	150	2x Average serving	257	32	5	12
		Meal Total	**257kcal**	**31.8g**	**4.8g**	**12.3g**
		Plan total	**3014kcal**	**363g**	**183g**	**92g**

16

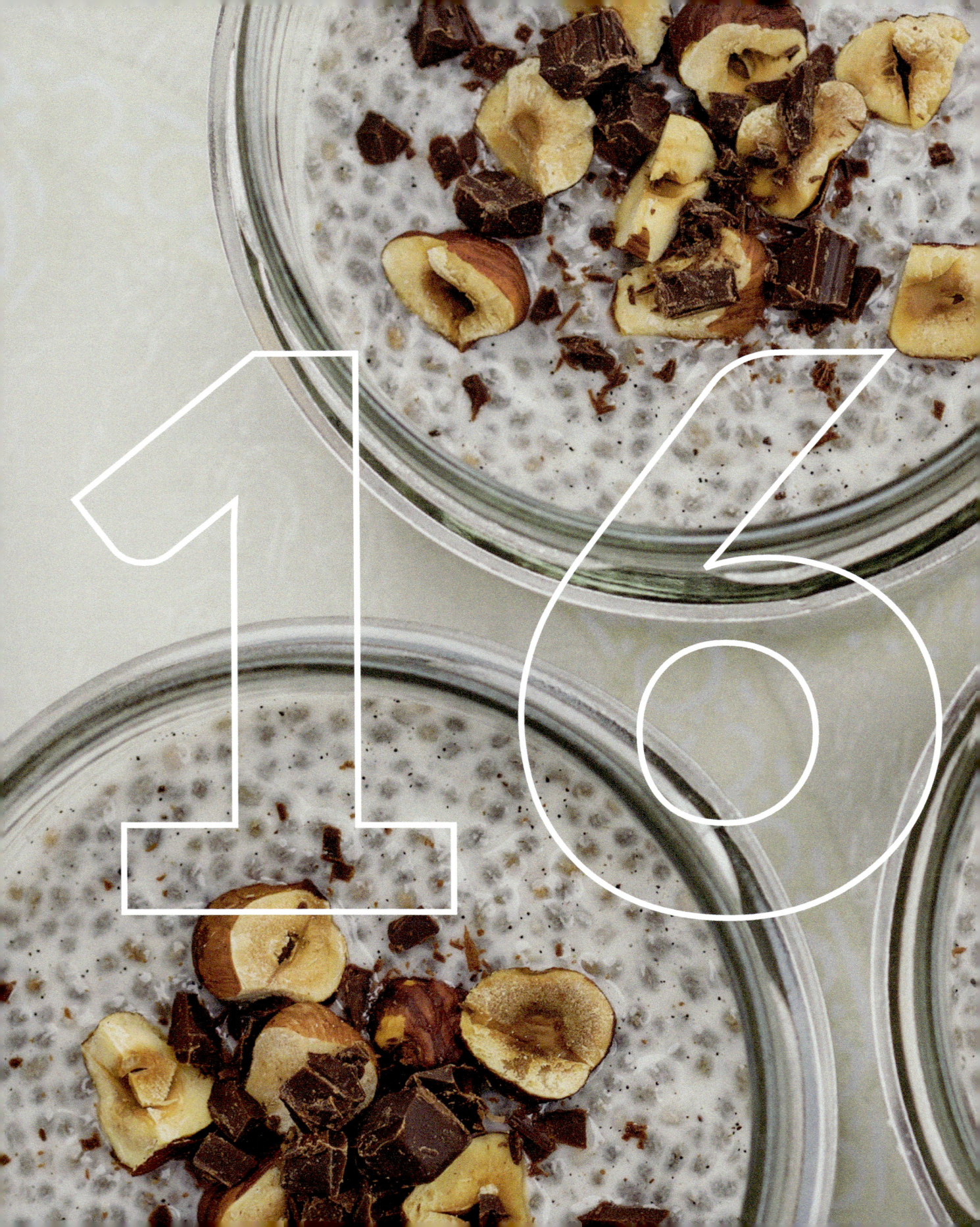

CHAPTER SIXTEEN
RECIPES

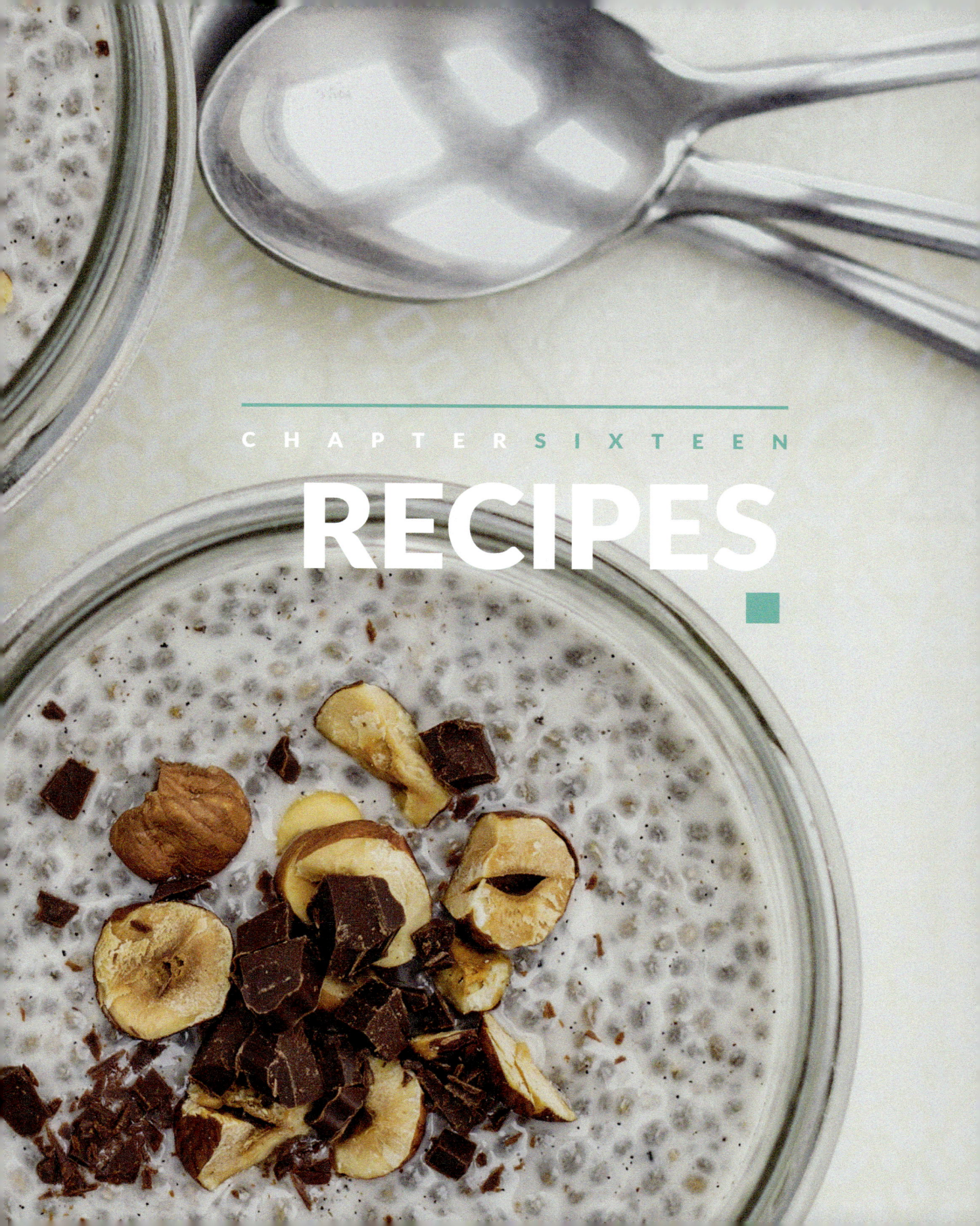

Overnight oats with chia seeds

An easy, tasty and filling breakfast choice to take to work or have when you get up. Experiment with different toppings to suit your preferences and goals.

Ingredients
1 tbsp of chia seeds
60g of oats
1 scoop of protein powder
160ml of semi skimmed milk or milk substitute
1 x small apple
2 tbsp of mixed berries

What to do
1. Mix the oats, protein, milk and chia seeds in a bowl and leave overnight in the fridge
2. Top with the berries and apple
3. Can also add dark chocolate!

Nutrition
Servings- 1
Kcals - 533 Carbs - 78 Fat - 10 Pro - 32

Breakfast smoothie

Another simple breakfast option ideal for those on the go. Simply throw your chosen ingredients in your smoothie maker and blitz.

Pick one of the following:
250-350ml regular milk
Coconut water
Milk substitution

Handful of one of the following
Spinach
Kale

1-2 of the following depending on kcal goals
Small handful of Blueberries
1 Apple, cored
1 Pear, cored
1 Peach/Nectarine, pitted

1 Banana
1 Mango
1 Kiwi

One scoop of protein
Whey/Soy/Vegan blend

One of the following
1 tbsp of nut butter – almond/cashew/peanut
1 tbsp of ground flaxseeds/sunflower seeds/chia seeds

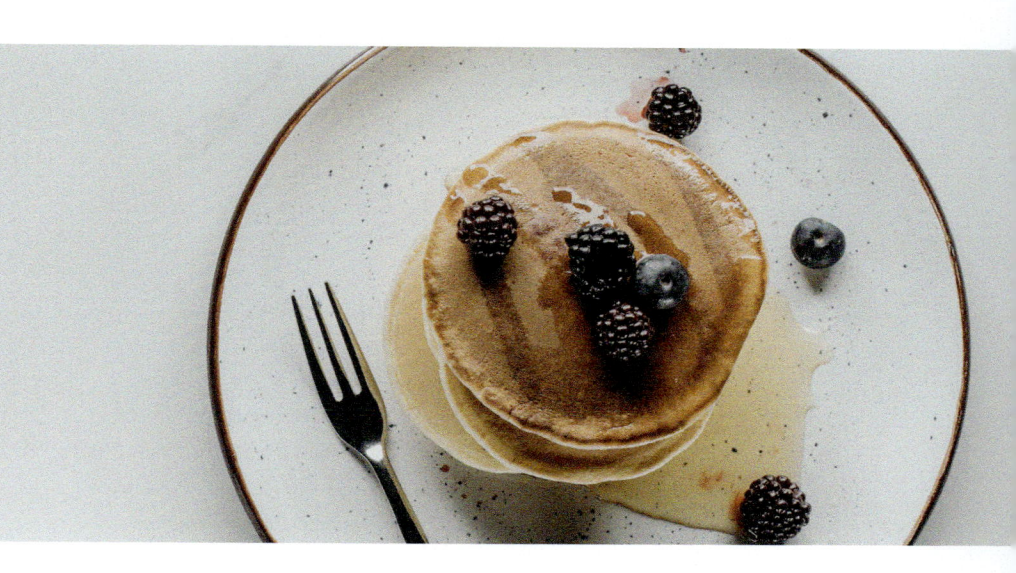

Protein pancakes

Ingredients

50g of oats
1 tbsp of ground flaxseeds
1 scoop of vanilla or chocolate whey
2 eggs, beaten
100ml milk
1 tsp butter
A handful of mixed berries
2 tbsp Greek yogurt

What to do

1. Mix the dry ingredients in a bowl
2. Add the beaten egg in a well in the centre of the oat mixture and enough of the milk to make the batter the consistency of single cream.
3. Leave to stand for 10 minutes
4. Take a frying pan and melt the butter
5. Pour a ladle of batter into the hot pan and tip to cover the surface
6. Bubbles will appear on the top surface of the pancake. Flip the pancake over when these bubbles start to pop
7. Slide out of the pan onto a warm plate and keep warm while making the rest
8. Serve with berries and Greek yogurt

Nutrition
Servings – 1
Kcals - 428 Carb - 41 Fat - 14 Pro - 35

Breakfast frittatas

One of our favourite "go-to" snacks, breakfasts and even lunches. Tasty (if you like eggs!), easy, high in protein and really filling too.

Ingredients	What to do
3 eggs	1. Beat eggs in a bowl
3 egg whites	2. Add veg to muffin tray
Handful of any veg (I like peas and spinach) – just play with what you like here	3. Add eggs to muffin tray (use butter/spray light/oil to grease -think kcals)
	4. Add (optional) cheese
60g of cheese	5. Bake (180c) for 12mins*

Nutrition
Servings – 1
Kcals - 428 Carb - 41 Fat - 14 Pro - 35

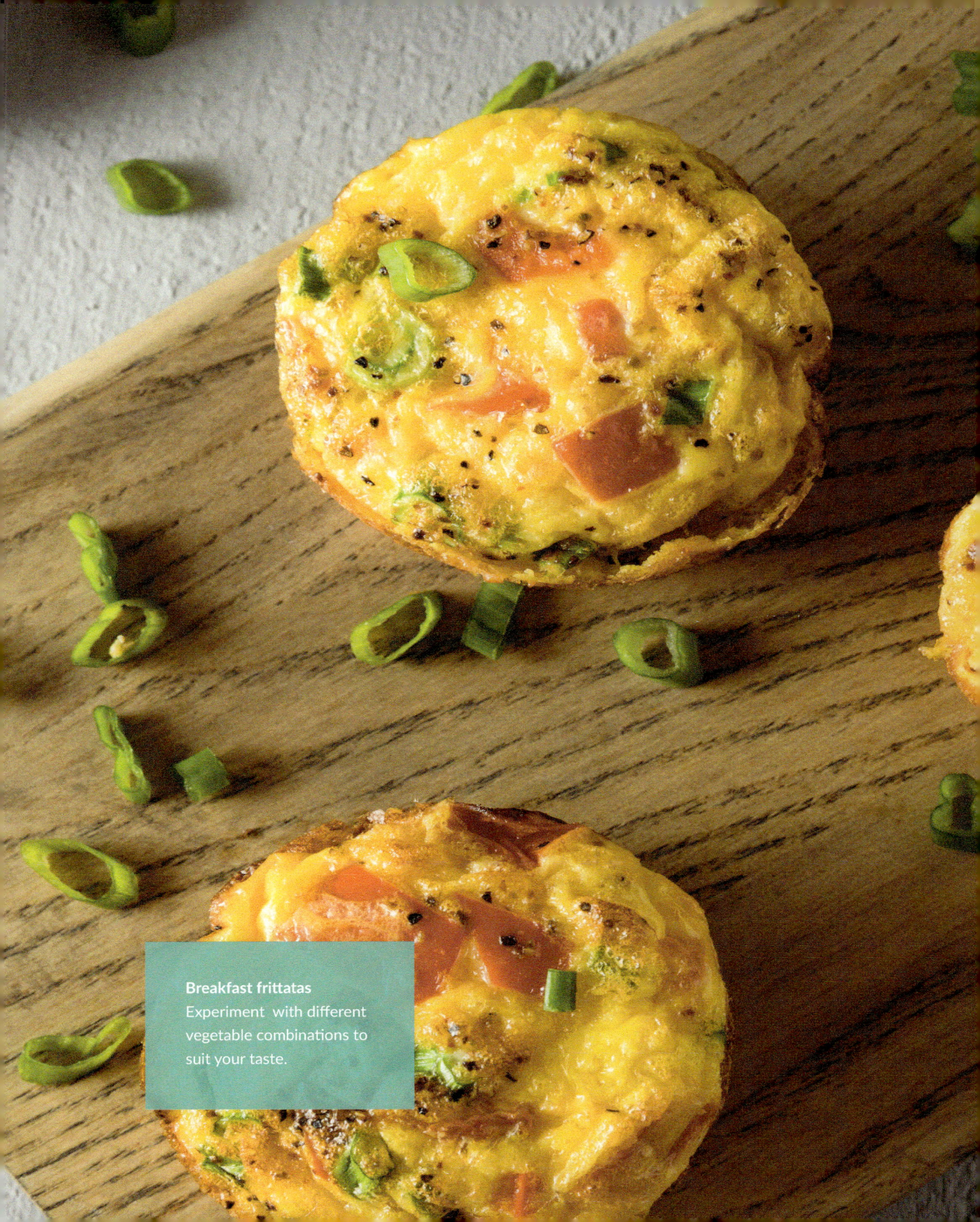

Breakfast frittatas
Experiment with different vegetable combinations to suit your taste.

Chicken and avocado flatbreads

Ingredients

2 x flat breads
1 x medium chicken breast
1/2 an avocado
3 x cherry tomatoes and sliced cucumber

What to do

1. Cook the chicken breast for 20mins at 180c
2. Carve a slit in the wholemeal flatbread or pitta
3. Slice the cooked chicken breast and season with salt and pepper.
4. Peel and core the avocado.
5. Mash avocado flesh in a bowl and stuff the pitta with it.
6. Add sliced chicken to the pitta.
7. Serve with a salad of your choice and season

Nutrition
Servings- 1
Kcals - 437 Carb - 37 Fat - 14 Pro - 40

Turkey meatballs and tzatziki in pitta

Ingredients

2 x pitta bread
For the meatballs
500g Turkey mince
1 x egg
45g of oats
30g of feta cheese
Handful of chopped parsley
Salt and pepper
For the tzatziki
50g of chopped cucumber
125g of 0% Greek yoghurt
1 tsp of lemon juice
Pinch black pepper

What to do

1. Mix together the ingredients for the meatballs in a large bowl. Make into ping pong balls.
2. Lightly spray the meatballs with a little olive oil, then bake for 10 – 12 minutes at 180c. After baking, allow them to slightly cool
3. Place the cucumber in a bowl and add the yogurt, pepper and lemon juice. Stir to combine.
4. Serve the meatballs in a pitta bread with the tzatziki and salad

Nutrition

For the meatballs:
Servings – Based on 4
Kcals - 263 Carb - 10 Fat - 8 Pro - 43

With 1 x pittas and tzatziki
Kcals - 446 Carb - 40 Fat - 13 Pro - 51
With 2 x pittas and tzatziki
Kcals - 626 Carb - 68 Fat - 14 Pro - 64

Build your protein salad

Salads don't need to be boring. There are hundreds of different ways to build these high protein lunches. Adjust your carbohydrate portions to match your needs.

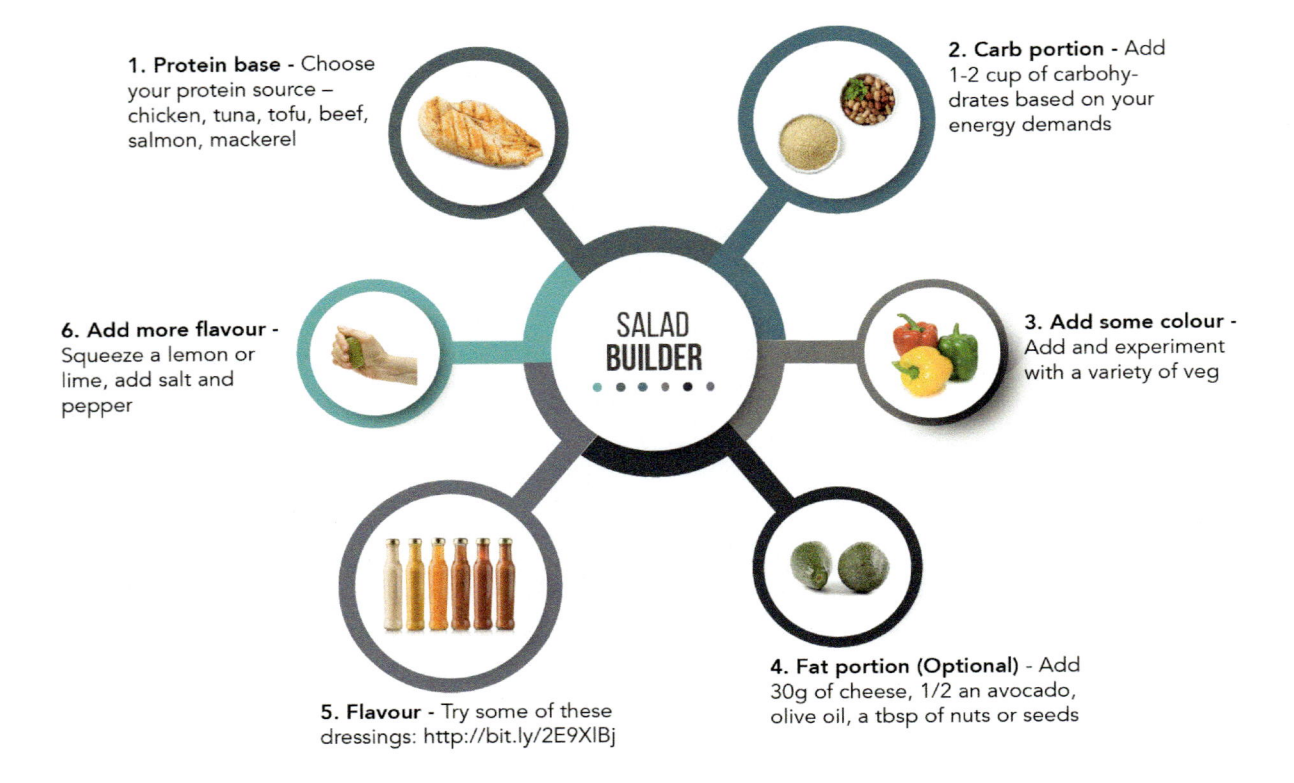

1. Protein base - Choose your protein source – chicken, tuna, tofu, beef, salmon, mackerel

2. Carb portion - Add 1-2 cup of carbohydrates based on your energy demands

6. Add more flavour - Squeeze a lemon or lime, add salt and pepper

SALAD BUILDER

3. Add some colour - Add and experiment with a variety of veg

5. Flavour - Try some of these dressings: http://bit.ly/2E9XlBj

4. Fat portion (Optional) - Add 30g of cheese, 1/2 an avocado, olive oil, a tbsp of nuts or seeds

Cajun chicken and sweet potato wedges

Ingredients

1 x chicken breast
2 x medium sweet potato
1 drizzle of olive oil
Paprika, cayenne pepper, cinnamon
Salt and pepper
Salad of choice

What to do

For the sweet potato wedges
1. Pre-heat the oven to 180C.
2. Cut the sweet potatoes into thick, even wedges – about an inch thick
3. Place the wedges onto a baking tray and cover them with olive oil, salt, paprika, cayenne pepper cinnamon.
4. Shake and mix together
5. Bake for about 45mins until soft. Shake every 15 mins

For the chicken
6. Cover the chicken with olive oil, cayenne pepper, paprika, chilli flakes and salt and pepper
7. Add to the oven with 20 minutes to go

Nutrition
Servings- 1
Kcals - 560 Carb - 59 Fat - 19 Pro - 39

Chermoula Chicken

Ingredients

For the chicken
Chicken, breast 1x medium fillet (130g)
1 tablespoon of olive oil
1/4 t-spoon of Cumin
1/4 t-spoon of Coriander
1 clove of Garlic
Lemon juice (not necessary)
1/2 t-spoon of Paprika
Pinch of Cayenne pepper
Salt and pepper
For the couscous:
100g of couscous, plain
1 x small apples (120g)
4 x cherry tomatoes (60g)
Red onion slices
20g of raisins
1/2-1 x small orange

What to do

1. To make the marinade, put the olive oil, cayenne pepper, fresh and ground coriander, cumin, garlic, lemon juice, paprika and parsley in a shallow dish and stir until smooth. Season with salt and pepper to taste.
2. Cut several slashes in each chicken breast. Add the chicken to the marinade and turn it until it is coated all over, rubbing the marinade into the slashes. Cover and chill for 2 hours.
3. Put a kettle on to boil. Put the couscous into a pan and pour 150 ml of boiling water over it. Cover and leave for 5 minutes to fluff up.
4. Meanwhile, stir the peaches, raisins, tomatoes, coriander and olive oil into the couscous. Adjust the seasoning to taste, cover and set aside.
5. Heat the grill to medium. Grill the chicken breasts for 3-4 minutes on each side, until the juices run clear when they are pierced with a knife. Carve them into slices and serve on top of the fruity couscous, garnished with a few sprigs of coriander.

Nutrition
Servings- 1
Kcals - 490 Carb - 68 Fat - 7 Pro - 45

Roasted veg

Ingredients

1 x handful of cherry tomatoes
1 x courgette
1 x aubergine
1 x pepper
1 x garlic clove
1 x red onion
150g of new potatoes
freshly ground black pepper
1 small bunch fresh rosemary (or dried)
1 small bunch fresh thyme (or dried)

What to do

1. Preheat the oven to 200°C/400°F/gas 6. Halve and deseed the pepper, then cut each half into 4 pieces. Peel the red onion and cut into wedge.
2. Halve the courgette lengthways then slice into 2cm chunks. Squash the garlic with you hand and add. Throw in cherry tomatoes. Chop the potatoes into small chunks or roast in separate tray.
3. Put all the veg in a roasting tray. Add salt and pepper, thyme and rosemary and drizzle it with olive oil.
4. Roast for around 45 minutes, or until soft.
5. Serve with anything from chicken to grilled meats or fish.

Nutrition
Servings- 3
Kcals - 172 Carb - 29 Fat - 5 Pro - 4

Slow cooked green Thai curry

Ingredients

2 skinless, boneless chicken breasts
2 tbsp green curry paste
1 tbsp ground cardamom
200ml tinned low fat coconut milk
1 red pepper, chopped
1 green pepper, chopped
2 medium sized carrots, chopped
2 onions, sliced
1 tbsp of fish sauce

What to do

1. 1 x lime, half juice and zest
2. Cook basmati rice (50g dry weight per person)
3. Switch the slow cooker to medium
4. Place all the ingredients into the slow cooker and give them good stir making sure the curry paste is evenly distributed
5. Cook for 5 hours on medium or 8 hours on low
6. Serve with basmati rice and lime wedges

Nutrition
Servings- 2
Kcals - 505 Carb - 66 Fat - 13 Pro - 28

Recipes

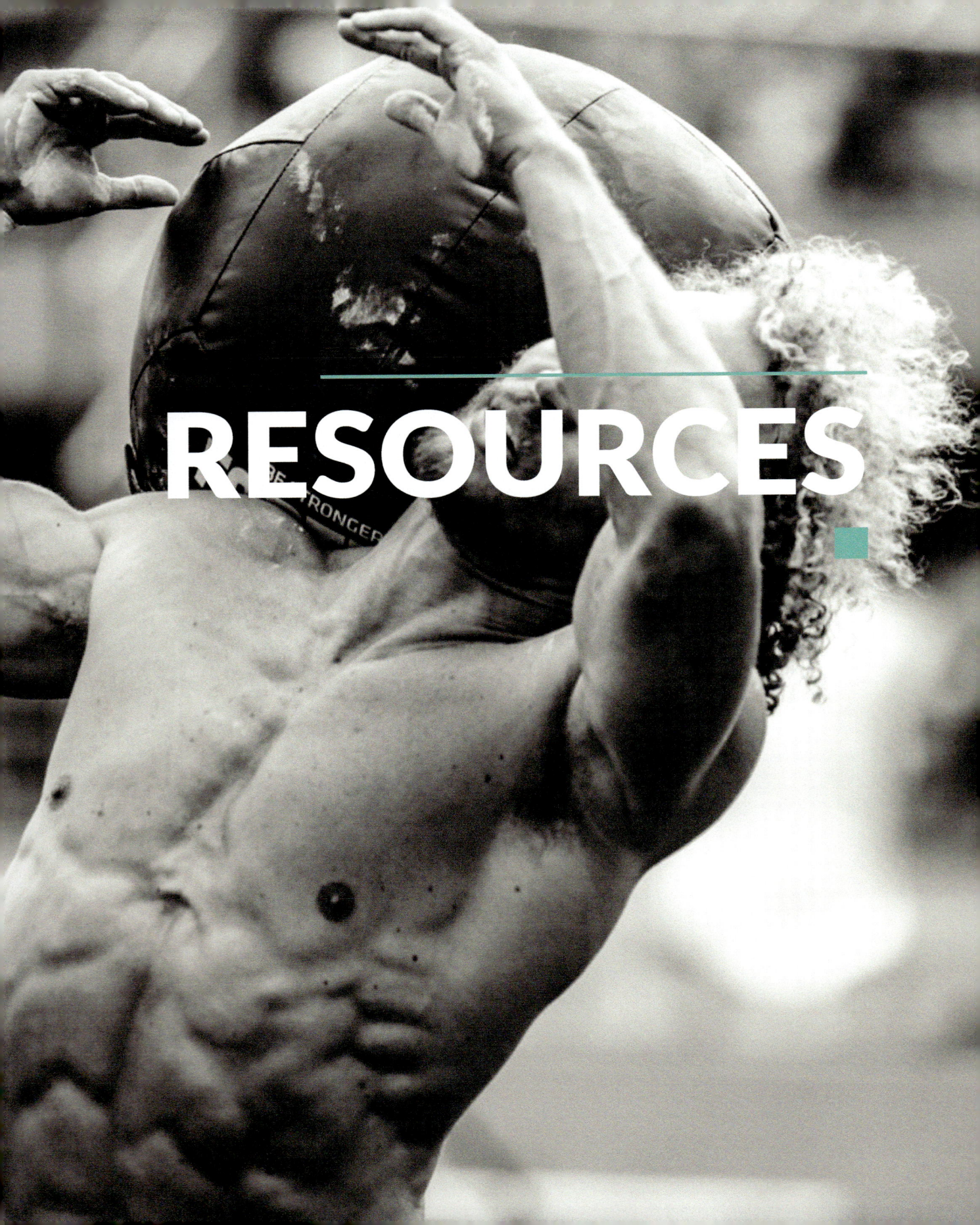

RESOURCES

Resource Section

For nutrition coaching, vist:

https://www.boxnutrition.co.uk/sign-up

For metabolic testing, visit:

https://www.boxnutrition.co.uk/metabolic-testing

To download your resource pack, visit:

www.boxnutrition.co.uk/fuellingresources

Your resource pack includes:

- *Macronutrient calculator*
- *Progress tracker*
- *Habit builder*
- *Meal planner*
- *Shopping list*
- *Snack guide*

For more nutrition support visit **www.boxnutrition.co.uk**

Other useful resources

Cost of getting lean infographic Precision Nutrition:

https://www.precisionnutrition.com/cost-of-getting-lean-infographic

Body fat calculator:

https://www.calculator.net/body-fat-calculator.html

The MET scale - Compendium of physical activities

Activity	Activity Specificity	METS
Cycling	Cycling, <10 mph, Leisure, to work or for pleasure (Taylor Code 115)	4
Cycling	Cycling, > 20 mph, racing, not drafting	15.8
Cycling	Cycling, 10-11.9 mph, Leisure, slow, light effort	6.8
Cycling	Cycling, 12 mph, seated, hands on brake hoods or bar drops, 80 rpm	8.5
Cycling	Cycling, 12-13.9 mph, Leisure, moderate effort	8
Cycling	Cycling, 14-15.9 mph, racing or Leisure, fast, vigorous effort	10
Cycling	Cycling, 16-19 mph, racing/not drafting or > 19 mph drafting, very fast, racing general	12
Cycling	Cycling, BMX	8.5
Cycling	Cycling, general	7.5
Cycling	Cycling, Leisure, 5.5 mph	3.5
Cycling	Cycling, Leisure, 9.4 mph	5.8
Cycling	Cycling, mountain, competitive, racing	16
Cycling	Cycling, mountain, general	8.5
Cycling	Cycling, mountain, general	7
Cycling	Cycling, mountain, uphill, vigorous	14
Cycling	Cycling, on dirt or farm road, moderate pace	5.8
Cycling	Cycling, to/from work, self selected pace	6.8
Conditioning Exercise	Rowing, stationary, 100 watts, moderate effort	7
Conditioning Exercise	Rowing, stationary, 150 watts, vigorous effort	8.5
Conditioning Exercise	Rowing, stationary, 200 watts, very vigorous effort	12
Conditioning Exercise	Cycling, stationary, 101-160 watts, vigorous effort	8.8
Conditioning Exercise	Cycling, stationary, 161-200 watts, vigorous effort	11
Conditioning Exercise	Cycling, stationary, 201-270 watts, very vigorous effort	14
Conditioning Exercise	Cycling, stationary, 30-50 watts, very light to light effort	3.5
Conditioning Exercise	Cycling, stationary, 51-89 watts, light-to-moderate effort	4.8
Conditioning Exercise	Cycling, stationary, 90-100 watts, moderate to vigorous effort	6.8
Conditioning Exercise	Cycling, stationary, RPM/Spin bike class	8.5
Conditioning Exercise	Calisthenics (e.g., push ups, sit ups, pull-ups, jumping jacks), vigorous effort	8
Conditioning Exercise	Calisthenics (e.g., push ups, sit ups, pull-ups, lunges), moderate effort	3.8
Conditioning Exercise	Calisthenics (e.g., situps, abdominal crunches), light effort	2.8
Conditioning Exercise	Calisthenics, light or moderate effort, general	3.5
Conditioning Exercise	Circuit training, including kettlebells, aerobic movement with little rest, vig intensity	8
Conditioning Exercise	circuit training, moderate effort	4.3
Conditioning Exercise	Elliptical trainer, moderate effort	5
Conditioning Exercise	Resistance training (weight lifting, free weights) powerlifting or bodybuilding, vigorous effort	6

Conditioning Exercise	Resistance training (weight) training, training, squats, slow or explosive effort	5
Inactivity	Sitting quietly, general	1.3
Leisure	Walking, 4.0 mph, level, firm surface, very brisk pace	5
Leisure	Walking, 4.5 mph, level, firm surface, very, very brisk	7
Leisure	Walking, 5.0 mph, level, firm surface	8.3
Leisure	Walking, 5.0 mph, uphill, 3% grade	9.8
Leisure	Walking, normal pace, plowed field or sand	4.5
Running	Running, 10 mph (6 min/mile)	14.5
Running	Running, 11 mph (5.5 min/mile)	16
Running	Running, 12 mph (5 min/mile)	19
Running	Running, 13 mph (4.6 min/mile)	19.8
Running	Running, 14 mph (4.3 min/mile)	23
Running	Running, 4 mph (13 min/mile)	6
Running	Running, 5 mph (12 min/mile)	8.3
Running	Running, 5.2 mph (11.5 min/mile)	9
Running	Running, 6 mph (10 min/mile)	9.8
Running	Running, 6.7 mph (9 min/mile)	10.5
Running	Running, 7 mph (8.5 min/mile)	11
Running	Running, 7.5 mph (8 min/mile)	11.5
Running	Running, 8 mph (7.5 min/mile)	11.8
Running	Running, 8.6 mph (7 min/mile)	12.3
Running	Running, 9 mph (6.5 min/mile)	12.8
Football	Competitive Football	10
Sports	Boxing (punching bag)	5.5
Sports	Boxing, sparring	7.8
Sports	Golf, general	4.8
Sports	Gymnastics	3.8
Sports	Rugby, union, team, competitive	8.3
Sports	Tennis, general	7.3
Swimming	Swimming laps, freestyle, fast, vigorous effort	9.8
Swimming	Swimming laps, freestyle, front crawl, slow, light or moderate effort	5.8
Swimming	Swimming, crawl, fast speed, ~75 yards/minute, vigorous effort	10
Swimming	Swimming, crawl, medium speed, ~50 yards/minute, vigorous effort	8.3
Yoga	Yoga	3.2

REFERENCES

Chapter 1 - What is functional fitness

1. McArdle, et al., 2010, p. 227. P165) McArdle, W., Katch, F. and Katch, V. (n.d.). Exercise physiology. 2010, p. 227. P165

2. Kenney, W., Wilmore, J. and Costill, D. (n.d.). Physiology of sport and exercise. p. 125)

3. MacLaren, D. and Morton, J. (2012). Biochemistry for sport and exercise metabolism. Chichester: Wiley-Blackwell.

4. Target Nutrition | Sports Dietitians | Brisbane & the Gold Coast. (2019). Target Nutrition Blog | Amie Cox's advice & tips | FREE!. [online] Available at: https://www.targetnutrition.com.au/blog/4-years-in-the-making-the-fourth-fittest-man-in-crossfit [Accessed 23 Jan. 2019].

Chapter 2

Energy demands

1. Kerksick, C., Wilborn, C., Roberts, M., Smith-Ryan, A., Kleiner, S., Jäger, R., Collins, R., Cooke, M., Davis, J., Galvan, E., Greenwood, M., Lowery, L., Wildman, R., Antonio, J. and Kreider, R. (2018). ISSN exercise & sports nutrition review update: research & recommendations. Journal of the International Society of Sports Nutrition, 15(1).

2. Burke, L. (2007). Practical sports nutrition. Leeds: Human Kinetics.

3. Kaewkannate, K. and Kim, S. (2016). A comparison of wearable fitness devices. BMC Public Health, 16(1).

4. Mountjoy, M., Sundgot-Borgen, J., Burke, L., Ackerman, K., Blauwet, C., Constantini, N., Lebrun, C., Lundy, B., Melin, A., Meyer, N., Sherman, R., Tenforde, A., Torstveit, M. and Budgett, R. (2018). International Olympic Committee (IOC) Consensus Statement on Relative Energy Deficiency in Sport (RED-S): 2018 Update. International Journal of Sport Nutrition and Exercise Metabolism, 28(4), pp.316-331.

5. Nutrition and Athletic Performance. (2016). Medicine & Science in Sports & Exercise® and in the Journal of the Academy of Nutrition and Dietetics, and the Canadian Journal of Dietetic Practice and Research., (Position Stand).

6. Garthe, I., Raastad, T., Refsnes, P., Koivisto, A. and Sundgot-Borgen, J. (2011). Effect of Two

Different Weight-Loss Rates on Body Composition and Strength and Power-Related Performance in Elite Athletes. International Journal of Sport Nutrition and Exercise Metabolism, 21(2), pp.97-104.

7. Boniface, A. (2019). #TrainBrave (via Passle). [online] Passle. Available at: http://insights.anna-boniface.com/post/102f7bo/trainbrave [Accessed 23 Jan. 2019].

Carbohydrates

8. Williams, C. and Rollo, I. (2015). Carbohydrate Nutrition and Team Sport Performance. Sports Medicine, 45(S1), pp.13-22.

9. Hawley, J. and Leckey, J. (2015). Carbohydrate Dependence During Prolonged, Intense Endurance Exercise. Sports Medicine, 45(S1), pp.5-12.

10. Kerksick, C., Wilborn, C., Roberts, M., Smith-Ryan, A., Kleiner, S., Jäger, R., Collins, R., Cooke, M., Davis, J., Galvan, E., Greenwood, M., Lowery, L., Wildman, R., Antonio, J. and Kreider, R. (2018). ISSN exercise & sports nutrition review update: research & recommendations. Journal of the International Society of Sports Nutrition, 15(1).

11. Escobar, K. and Morales, J. (2015). The Effect Of Carbohydrate Intake On Crossfit

12. Burke, L., Ross, M., Garvican-Lewis, L., Welvaert, M., Heikura, I., Forbes, S., Mirtschin, J., Cato, L., Strobel, N., Sharma, A. and Hawley, J. (2017). Low carbohydrate, high fat diet impairs exercise economy and negates the performance benefit from intensified training in elite race walkers. The Journal of Physiology, 595(9), pp.2785-2807.

13. Hargreaves, M., Hawley, J. and Jeukendrup, A. (2004). Pre-exercise carbohydrate and fat ingestion: effects on metabolism and performance. Journal of Sports Sciences, 22(1), pp.31-38.

14. Hawley JA, Palmer GS, Noakes TD. Effects of 3 days of carbohydrate supplementation on muscle glycogen content and utilisation during a 1-h cycling performance. Eur J Appl Physiol Occup Physiol 75(5):407-12, 1997.

15. Temesi, J., Johnson, N., Raymond, J., Burdon, C. and O'Connor, H. (2011). Carbohydrate Ingestion during Endurance Exercise Improves Performance in Adults. Journal of Nutrition, 141(5), pp.890-897.

16. Burke, L., Hawley, J., Wong, S. and Jeukendrup, A. (2011). Carbohydrates for training and competition. Journal of Sports Sciences, 29(sup1), pp.S17-S27.

17. Thomas, D., Erdman, K. and Burke, L. (2016). Position of the Academy of Nutrition and

Dietetics, Dietitians of Canada, and the American College of Sports Medicine: Nutrition and Athletic Performance. Journal of the Academy of Nutrition and Dietetics, 116(3), pp.501-528.

18. Cermak, N. and van Loon, L. (2013). The Use of Carbohydrates During Exercise as an Ergogenic Aid. Sports Medicine, 43(11), pp.1139-1155.

19. Chakravarthy, M.V., and F.W. Booth (2004). Eating, exercise, and "thrifty" genotypes: connecting the dots toward an evolutionary understanding of modern chronic diseases. J. Appl. Physiol. 96:3-10.

20. Phinney, S., Bistrian, B., Wolfe, R. and Blackburn, G. (1983). The human metabolic response to chronic ketosis without caloric restriction: Physical and biochemical adaptation. Metabolism, 32(8), pp.757-768.

21. Volek, J., Freidenreich, D., Saenz, C., Kunces, L., Creighton, B., Bartley, J., Davitt, P., Munoz, C., Anderson, J., Maresh, C., Lee, E., Schuenke, M., Aerni, G., Kraemer, W. and Phinney, S. (2016). Metabolic characteristics of keto-adapted ultra-endurance runners. Metabolism, 65(3), pp.100-110.

22. Webster, C., Noakes, T., Chacko, S., Swart, J., Kohn, T. and Smith, J. (2016). Gluconeogenesis during endurance exercise in cyclists habituated to a long-term low carbohydrate high-fat diet. The Journal of Physiology, 594(15), pp.4389-4405.

23. Burke, L., Kiens, B. and Ivy, J. (2004). Carbohydrates and fat for training and recovery. Journal of Sports Sciences, 22(1), pp.15-30.

24. Burke, L. (2015). Re-Examining High-Fat Diets for Sports Performance: Did We Call the 'Nail in the Coffin' Too Soon?. Sports Med, 45(S1), pp.33-49.

25. Hawley, J. and Leckey, J. (2015). Carbohydrate Dependence During Prolonged, Intense Endurance Exercise. Sports Medicine, 45(S1), pp.5-12.

26. Currell, K. (2016). Performance Nutrition. Crowood.

27. Cholewa, J., Newmire, D. and Zanchi, N. (2018). Carbohydrate Restriction: Friend or Foe of Resistance-Based Exercise Performance?. Nutrition.

28. MacLaren, D. and Morton, J. (2012). Biochemistry for sport and exercise metabolism. Chichester: Wiley-Blackwell. P 153

29. Morton, J. (2016). Fasted training. [online] Runner's World. Available at: http://www.runnersworld.co.uk/health/fasted-training/10235.html [Accessed 28 Jan. 2019].

30. Hawley, J., Lundby, C., Cotter, J. and Burke, L. (2018). Maximizing Cellular Adaptation to Endurance Exercise in Skeletal Muscle. Cell Metabolism, 27(5), pp.962-976.

31. Impey, S., Hearris, M., Hammond, K., Bartlett, J., Louis, J., Close, G. and Morton, J. (2018). Fuel for the Work Required: A Theoretical Framework for Carbohydrate Periodization and the Glycogen Threshold Hypothesis. Sports Medicine, 48(5), pp.1031-1048.

32. Bannock, L., Robinson, S. and Owens, D. (2016). Guru Performance Position Stand #1 - Fasted Training & Body Composition. 1st ed. [ebook] London: NA. Available at: http://guruperformance.com/ [Accessed 26 Jan. 2019].

33. Iwayama, K., Kurihara, R., Nabekura, Y., Kawabuchi, R., Park, I., Kobayashi, M., Ogata, H., Kayaba, M., Satoh, M. and Tokuyama, K. (2015). Exercise Increases 24-h Fat Oxidation Only When It Is Performed Before Breakfast. EBioMedicine, 2(12), pp.2003-2009.

34. Amorim Andrade-Souza, V., Ghiarone, T., Sansonio, A., Augusto Santos Silva, K. and Tomazini, F. (2019). Exercise twice-a-day potentiates skeletal muscle signalling responses associated with mitochondrial biogenesis in humans, which are independent of lowered muscle glycogen content.

35. Hulston, C, Venables, M, Mann, C, Martin, C, Philp, A, Baar, K and Jeukendrup, A. (2010). Training with Low Muscle Glycogen Enhances Fat Metabolism in Well-Trained Cyclists. Medicine & Science in Sports & Exercise, 42(11), pp.2046-2055.

36. Yeo, W., Carey, A., Burke, L., Spriet, L. and Hawley, J. (2011). Fat adaptation in well-trained athletes: effects on cell metabolism. Applied Physiology, Nutrition, and Metabolism, 36(1), pp.12-22.

37. Kasper, A., Cocking, S., Cockayne, M., Barnard, M., Tench, J., Parker, L., McAndrew, J., Langan-Evans, C., Close, G. and Morton, J. (2015). Carbohydrate mouth rinse and caffeine improves high-intensity interval running capacity when carbohydrate restricted. European Journal of Sport Science, 16(5), pp.560-568.

38. Venkatraman, J. and Pendergast, D. (2002). Effect of Dietary Intake on Immune Function in Athletes. Sports Medicine, 32(5), pp.323-337.

39. Helms, E., Aragon, A. and Fitschen, P. (2014). Evidence-based recommendations for natural bodybuilding contest preparation: nutrition and supplementation. Journal of the International Society of Sports Nutrition, 11(1).

40. Gardner, C.D., Trepanowski, J.F., Del Gobbo, L.C., Hauser, M.E., Rigdon, J., Ioannidis,

J.P.A., Desai, M. and King, A.C. (2018) 'Effect of Low-Fat vs Low-Carbohydrate Diet on 12-Month Weight Loss in Overweight Adults and the Association With Genotype Pattern or Insulin Secretion: The DIETFITS Randomized Clinical Trial', Jama, 319(7), pp. 667-679.

41. Ye, E., Chacko, S., Chou, E., Kugizaki, M. and Liu, S. (2012). Greater Whole-Grain Intake Is Associated with Lower Risk of Type 2 Diabetes, Cardiovascular Disease, and Weight Gain. Journal of Nutrition, 142(7), pp.1304-1313.

42. Flight, I. and Clifton, P. (2006). Cereal grains and legumes in the prevention of coronary heart disease and stroke: a review of the literature. European Journal of Clinical Nutrition, 60(10), pp.1145-1159.

43. CyclingTips. (2019). Fueling Team Sky's nutrition for the Tour de France | CyclingTips. [online] Available at: https://cyclingtips.com/2016/07/fueling-for-the-tour-de-france-with-team-skys-head-of-nutrition/ [Accessed 14 Jan. 2019]

Protein

44. Phillips 2016 (Phillips, S., Chevalier, S. and Leidy, H. (2016). Protein "requirements" beyond the RDA: implications for optimizing health. Applied Physiology, Nutrition, and Metabolism, 41(5), pp.565-572.)

45. Jager, R., Kerksick, C.M., Campbell, B.I., Cribb, P.J., Wells., SKWiatT, T.M., Purpura, M., Ziegenfuss, T.N., Ferrando, A.A., Arent, S.M., Smith-Ryan, A.E., Stout, J.R., Arciero, P.J., Ormsbee, M.J., Taylor, L.W., Wilborn, C.D., Kalman, D.S., Krieder, R.B., Willoughby, D.S., Hoffman, J.R., Krzykowski, J.L. and Antonio, J., 2017. International Society of Sports Nutrition Position Stand: protein and exercise. Journal of the International Society of Sports Nutrition, 14, pp. 20-017-0177-8. eCollection 2017.

46. Mettle, S., Mitchell, N. and Tipton, K. (2010). Increased Protein Intake Reduces Lean Body Mass Loss during Weight Loss in Athletes. Medicine & Science in Sports & Exercise, 42(2), pp.326-337.

47. Phillips, S. and Van Loon, L. (2011). Dietary protein for athletes: From requirements to optimum adaptation. Journal of Sports Sciences, 29(sup1), pp.S29-S38.

48. Tipton, K. (2015). Nutritional Support for Exercise-Induced Injuries. Sports Medicine, 45(S1), pp.93-104.

49. Phillips, S. (2012). Dietary protein requirements and adaptive advantages in athletes. British Journal of Nutrition, 108(S2), pp.S158-S167.

Fat

50. Bird, S. (2010). Strength Nutrition: Maximizing Your Anabolic Potential. Strength and Conditioning Journal, 32(4), pp.80-86.

51. Venkatraman, J., Leddy, J. and Pendergast, D. (2000). Dietary fats and immune status in athletes: clinical implications. Medicine & Science in Sports & Exercise, 32(Supplement), pp.S389-S395.

52. Stellingwerff, T., Maughan, R. and Burke, L. (2011). Nutrition for power sports: Middle-distance running, track cycling, rowing, canoeing/kayaking, and swimming. Journal of Sports Sciences, 29(sup1), pp.S79-S89.

53. Schwingshackl, L. and Hoffmann, G. (2013). Long-term effects of low-fat diets either low or high in protein on cardiovascular and metabolic risk factors: a systematic review and meta-analysis. Nutrition Journal, 12(1).

Should we be going Keto

55 J Int Soc Sports Nutr. 2016 Jan 16;13:3. doi: 10.1186/s12970-016-0114-2. eCollection 2016. The effects of a high protein diet on indices of health and body composition--a crossover trial in resistance-trained men. Antonio J, Ellerbroek A, Silver T, Vargas L, Peacock CJ Int Soc Sports Nutr. 2016 Jan 16;13:3. doi: 10.1186/s12970-016-0114-2. eCollection 2016.

56 Effects of dietary protein intake on body composition changes after weight loss in older adults: a systematic review and meta-analysis. Jung Eun Kim, Lauren E. O'Connor, Laura P. Sands, Mary B. Slebodnik, Wayne W.Campbell. Nutrition Reviews Mar 2016, 74 (3) 210-224; DOI: 10.1093/nutrit/nuv065

57 Palmer BF, Henrich WL. "Carbohydrate and insulin metabolism in chronic kidney disease". UpToDate, Inc.

58 Volek JS, e. (2016). Comparison of a very low-carbohydrate and low-fat diet on fasting lipids, LDL subclasses, insulin resistance, and postprandial lipemic responses in... - PubMed - NCBI. [online] Ncbi.nlm.nih.gov. Available at: http://www.ncbi.nlm.nih.gov/pubmed/15047685 [Accessed 14 Oct. 2016].

59 Samaha F, Foster GD, Makris AP, Low-carbohydrate diets, obesity, and metabolic risk factors for cardiovascular disease. Curr Atheroscler Rep.2007 Dec;9(6):441-7.

60 Chang, C., Borer, K. and Lin, P. (2017). Low-Carbohydrate-High-Fat Diet: Can it Help Exercise Performance?. Journal of Human Kinetics, 56(1), pp.81-92.

61 Burke, L., Hawley, J., Jeukendrup, A., Morton, J., Stellingwerff, T. and Maughan, R. (2018). Toward a Common Understanding of Diet–Exercise Strategies to Manipulate Fuel Availability for Training and Competition Preparation in Endurance Sport. International Journal of Sport Nutrition and Exercise Metabolism, 28(5), pp.451-463.

62 Hall, K.D., Guo, J., Obesity energetics: body weight regulation and the effects of diet composition. Gastroenterology, 2017. 152(7): p. 1718–27.

63 Sci-Fit. (2019). Adhering to the Ketogenic Diet - Is it Easy or Hard? (Research Review) • Sci-Fit. [online] Available at: https://sci-fit.net/adhere-ketogenic-diet/ [Accessed 14 Jan. 2019].

Micronutrients

64 Whiting, S. and Barabash, W. (2006). Dietary Reference Intakes for the micronutrients: considerations for physical activity. Applied Physiology, Nutrition, and Metabolism, 31(1), pp.80-85.

65 Pojednic, R. and Ceglia, L. (2014). The Emerging Biomolecular Role of Vitamin D in Skeletal Muscle. Exercise and Sport Sciences Reviews, 42(2), pp.76-81.

66 Tomlinson, P., Joseph, C. and Angioi, M. (2015). Effects of vitamin D supplementation on upper and lower body muscle strength levels in healthy individuals. A systematic review with meta-analysis. Journal of Science and Medicine in Sport, 18(5), pp.575-580.

67 Ogan, D. and Pritchett, K. (2013). Vitamin D and the Athlete: Risks, Recommendations, and Benefits. Nutrients, 5(6), pp.1856-1868.

68 Vitamin D and Health. (2016). Scientific advisory Committee on Nutrition.

69 Vitale, K., Hueglin, S. and Broad, E. (2017). Tart Cherry Juice in Athletes. Current Sports Medicine Reports, 16(4), pp.230-239.

70 Gleeson, M. (2005). Assessing immune function changes in exercise and diet intervention studies. Current Opinion in Clinical Nutrition and Metabolic Care, 8(5), pp.511-515.

71 Woolf, K. and Manore, M. (2006). B-Vitamins and Exercise: Does Exercise Alter Requirements?. International Journal of Sport Nutrition and Exercise Metabolism, 16(5), pp.453-484.

72 Gabel, K. (2006). Special Nutritional Concerns for the Female Athlete. Current Sports Medicine Reports, 5(4), pp.187-191.

73 Gleeson, M. and Williams, C. (2013) 'Intense exercise training and immune function', Nestle Nutrition Institute workshop series, 76, pp. 39-50. doi: 10.1159/000350254 [doi].

74 Nieman, D.C. (1999) 'Nutrition, exercise, and immune system function', Clinics in sports

medicine, 18(3), pp. 537-548. doi: S0278-5919(05)70167-8 [pii].

Chapter 3 – Fuelling your workouts

1. Kerksick, C., Wilborn, C., Roberts, M., Smith-Ryan, A., Kleiner, S., Jäger, R., Collins, R., Cooke, M., Davis, J., Galvan, E., Greenwood, M., Lowery, L., Wildman, R., Antonio, J. and Kreider, R. (2018). ISSN exercise & sports nutrition review update: research & recommendations. Journal of the International Society of Sports Nutrition, 15(1).

2. Temple, N. (2012). Nutritional health. New York: Springer, pp.207-235.

3. Chryssanthopoulos, C. and Williams, C. (1997). Pre-Exercise Carbohydrate Meal and Endurance Running Capacity when Carbohydrates are Ingested During Exercise. International Journal of Sports Medicine, 18(07), pp.543-548.

4. Wright, D., Sherman, W. and Dernbach, A. (1991). Carbohydrate feedings before, during, or in combination improve cycling endurance performance. Journal of Applied Physiology, 71(3), pp.1082-1088.

5. Burke, L., Hawley, J., Wong, S. and Jeukendrup, A. (2011). Carbohydrates for training and competition. Journal of Sports Sciences, 29(sup1), pp.S17-S27.

6. Cermak, N. and van Loon, L. (2013). The Use of Carbohydrates During Exercise as an Ergogenic Aid. Sports Medicine, 43(11), pp.1139-1155.

7. Gatorade Sports Science Institute. (2019). Dietary Carbohydrate & Performance of Brief, Intense Exercise. [online] Available at: https://www.gssiweb.org/sports-science-exchange/article/sse-79-dietary-carbohydrate-performance-of-brief-intense-exercise [Accessed 28 Jan. 2019].

8. Nutrition and Athletic Performance. (2016). Medicine & Science in Sports & Exercise® and in the Journal of the Academy of Nutrition and Dietetics, and the Canadian Journal of Dietetic Practice and Research., (Position Stand).

9. Hargreaves, M., Hawley, J. and Jeukendrup, A. (2004). Pre-exercise carbohydrate and fat ingestion: effects on metabolism and performance. Journal of Sports Sciences, 22(1), pp.31-38.

10. Ormsbee, M., Bach, C. and Baur, D. (2014). Pre-Exercise Nutrition: The Role of Macronutrients, Modified Starches and Supplements on Metabolism and Endurance Performance. Nutrients, 6(5), pp.1782-1808.

11. Burke, L., Hawley, J., Wong, S. and Jeukendrup, A. (2011). Carbohydrates for training and competition. Journal of Sports Sciences, 29(sup1), pp.S17-S27.

12. Jamurtas, A., Tofas, T., Fatouros, I., Nikolaidis, M., Paschalis, V., Yfanti, C., Raptis, S. and Koutedakis, Y. (2011). The effects of low and high glycemic index foods on exercise performance and beta-endorphin responses. Journal of the International Society of Sports Nutrition, 8(1).

13. Maughan, R. and Noakes, T. (1991). Fluid Replacement and Exercise Stress. Sports Medicine, 12(1), pp.16-31.

14. Jentjens, R. L., et al. (2004). Oxidation of combined ingestion of glucose and fructose during exercise." J Appl Physiol 96(4): 1277-1284.

15. Currell, K. and A. E. Jeukendrup (2008). Superior endurance performance with ingestion of multiple transportable carbohydrates." Med Sci Sports Exerc 40(2): 275-281.

16. Phillips, S., Sproule, J. and Turner, A. (2011). Carbohydrate Ingestion during Team Games Exercise. Sports Medicine, 41(7), pp.559-585.

17. Currell, K., Conway, S. and Jeukendrup, A. (2009). Carbohydrate Ingestion Improves Performance of a New Reliable Test of Soccer Performance. International Journal of Sport Nutrition and Exercise Metabolism, 19(1), pp.34-46.

18. Saunders, M., Luden, N. and Herrick, J. (2007). Consumption of an Oral Carbohydrate-Protein Gel Improves Cycling Endurance and Prevents Postexercise Muscle Damage. The Journal of Strength and Conditioning Research, 21(3), p.678.

19. Zawadzki, K., Yaspelkis, B. and Ivy, J. (1992). Carbohydrate-protein complex increases the rate of muscle glycogen storage after exercise. Journal of Applied Physiology, 72(5), pp.1854-1859.

20. Currell, K. (2016). Performance Nutrition. Crowood.

21. Aragon, A. and Schoenfeld, B. (2013). Nutrient timing revisited: is there a post-exercise anabolic window?. Journal of the International Society of Sports Nutrition, 10(1).

22. Heaton, L., Davis, J., Rawson, E., Nuccio, R., Witard, O., Stein, K., Baar, K., Carter, J. and Baker, L. (2017). Selected In-Season Nutritional Strategies to Enhance Recovery for Team Sport Athletes: A Practical Overview. Sports Medicine, 47(11), pp.2201-2218.

Chapter 4 – Supplements

1. Kreider, R., Kalman, D., Antonio, J., Ziegenfuss, T., Wildman, R., Collins, R., Candow, D., Kleiner, S., Almada, A. and Lopez, H. (2017). International Society of Sports Nutrition position stand: safety and efficacy of creatine supplementation in exercise, sport, and medicine. Journal of the International Society of Sports Nutrition, 14(1).

2. McNaughton, L., Dalton, B. and Tarr, J. (1998). The effects of creatine supplementation on high-intensity exercise performance in elite performers. European Journal of Applied Physiology, 78(3), pp.236-240.

3. Nutrition and Athletic Performance. (2016). Medicine & Science in Sports & Exercise® and in the Journal of the Academy of Nutrition and Dietetics, and the Canadian Journal of Dietetic Practice and Research., (Position Stand).

4. Cooper, R., Naclerio, F., Allgrove, J. and Jimenez, A. (2012). Creatine supplementation with specific view to exercise/sports performance: an update. Journal of the International Society of Sports Nutrition, 9(1), p.33.

5. Hultman E, et al. Muscle creatine loading in men. J Appl Physiol (1985). 1996;81(1):232–

6. Lancha Junior, A., de Salles Painelli, V., Saunders, B. and Artioli, G. (2015). Nutritional Strategies to Modulate Intracellular and Extracellular Buffering Capacity During High-Intensity Exercise. Sports Medicine, 45(S1), pp.71-81.

7. Saunders, B., Elliott-Sale, K., Artioli, G., Swinton, P., Dolan, E., Roschel, H., Sale, C. and Gualano, B. (2016). β-alanine supplementation to improve exercise capacity and performance: a systematic review and meta-analysis. British Journal of Sports Medicine, 51(8), pp.658-669.

8. Goldstein, E., Ziegenfuss, T., Kalman, D., Kreider, R., Campbell, B., Wilborn, C., Taylor, L., Willoughby, D., Stout, J., Graves, B., Wildman, R., Ivy, J., Spano, M., Smith, A. and Antonio, J. (2010). International society of sports nutrition position stand: caffeine and performance. Journal of the International Society of Sports Nutrition, 7(1), p.5.

9. Graham, T. E. & Spriet, L. L. (1991) Performance and metabolic responses to a high caffeine dose during prolonged exercise. J Appl Physiol, 71, 2292-2298.

10. Graham, T. E. & Spriet, L. L.. (1995) Metabolic, catecholamine, and exercise performance responses to various doses of caffeine. J Appl Physiol, 78, 867-874.

11. Smith-Ryan, A. And Antonio, J.Sports Nutrition and performance enhancing supplements In-text: (Smith-Ryan and Antonio) Bibliography: Smith-Ryan, Abbie, and Jose Antonio. Sports Nutrition And Performance Enhancing Supplements. New York: Linus Leanring, 2013. Print.

12. Hodgson, Adrian B., Rebecca K. Randell, and Asker E. Jeukendrup. 'The Metabolic And Performance Effects Of Caffeine Compared To Coffee During Endurance Exercise'. PLoS ONE 8.4 (2013): e59561. Web. 5 Aug. 2015.

13. Maughan, R., Burke, L., Dvorak, J., Larson-Meyer, D., Peeling, P., Phillips, S., Rawson, E.,

Walsh, N., Garthe, I., Geyer, H., Meeusen, R., van Loon, L., Shirreffs, S., Spriet, L., Stuart, M., Vernec, A., Currell, K., Ali, V., Budgett, R., Ljungqvist, A., Mountjoy, M., Pitsiladis, Y., Soligard, T., Erdener, U. and Engebretsen, L. (2018). IOC consensus statement: dietary supplements and the high-performance athlete. British Journal of Sports Medicine, 52(7), pp.439-455.

14. Kramer, S., Baur, D., Spicer, M., Vukovich, M. and Ormsbee, M. (2016). The effect of six days of dietary nitrate supplementation on performance in trained CrossFit athletes. Journal of the International Society of Sports Nutrition, 13(1).

15. Kerksick, C., Wilborn, C., Roberts, M., Smith-Ryan, A., Kleiner, S., Jäger, R., Collins, R., Cooke, M., Davis, J., Galvan, E., Greenwood, M., Lowery, L., Wildman, R., Antonio, J. and Kreider, R. (2018). ISSN exercise & sports nutrition review update: research & recommendations. Journal of the International Society of Sports Nutrition, 15(1).

16. Hoon, M., Jones, A., Johnson, N., Blackwell, J., Broad, E., Lundy, B., Rice, A. and Burke, L. (2014). The Effect of Variable Doses of Inorganic Nitrate-Rich Beetroot Juice on Simulated 2000-m Rowing Performance in Trained Athletes. International Journal of Sports Physiology and Performance, 9(4), pp.615-620.

17. Vitale, K., Hueglin, S. and Broad, E. (2017). Tart Cherry Juice in Athletes. Current Sports Medicine Reports, 16(4), pp.230-239.

18. Martinez, N., Campbell, B., Franek, M., Buchanan, L. and Colquhoun, R. (2016). The effect of acute pre-workout supplementation on power and strength performance. Journal of the International Society of Sports Nutrition, 13(1).

19. Pérez-Guisado, J. and Jakeman, P. (2010). Citrulline Malate Enhances Athletic Anaerobic Performance and Relieves Muscle Soreness. Journal of Strength and Conditioning Research, 24(5), pp.1215-1222.

Part 2

1. Helms, E., Aragon, A. and Fitschen, P. (2014). Evidence-based recommendations for natural bodybuilding contest preparation: nutrition and supplementation. Journal of the International Society of Sports Nutrition, 11(1).

2. Garthe, I., Raastad, T., Refsnes, P., Koivisto, A. and Sundgot-Borgen, J. (2011). Effect of Two Different Weight-Loss Rates on Body Composition and Strength and Power-Related Performance in Elite Athletes. International Journal of Sport Nutrition and Exercise Metabolism, 21(2), pp.97-104.

3. Helms, E. and Morgan, A. (2017). The Muscle & Strength Pyramid - Training.

4. Longland TM, e. (2019). Higher compared with lower dietary protein during an energy deficit combined with intense exercise promotes greater lean mass gain and fat mass los... - PubMed - NCBI. [online] Ncbi.nlm.nih.gov. Available at: https://www.ncbi.nlm.nih.gov/pubmed/26817506 [Accessed 10 Feb. 2019].

5. Aragon, A., Schoenfeld, B., Wildman, R., Kleiner, S., VanDusseldorp, T., Taylor, L., Earnest, C., Arciero, P., Wilborn, C., Kalman, D., Stout, J., Willoughby, D., Campbell, B., Arent, S., Bannock, L., Smith-Ryan, A. and Antonio, J. (2017). International society of sports nutrition position stand: diets and body composition. Journal of the International Society of Sports Nutrition, 14(1).

Tips for improving sleep

6. Fetveit, A., Skjerve, A. and Bjorvatn, B. (2003). Bright light treatment improves sleep in institutionalised elderly?an open trial. International Journal of Geriatric Psychiatry, 18(6), pp.520-526.

7. Drake, C., Roehrs, T., Shambroom, J. and Roth, T. (2013). Caffeine Effects on Sleep Taken 0, 3, or 6 Hours before Going to Bed. Journal of Clinical Sleep Medicine.

8. Van Dongen, H. and Dinges, D. (2003). Investigating the interaction between the homeostatic and circadian processes of sleep-wake regulation for the prediction of waking neurobehavioural performance. Journal of Sleep Research, 12(3), pp.181-187.

9. Autonomic Stress Tests in Obstructive Sleep Apnea Syndrome and Snoring. (1992). Sleep.

10. Kanda, K., Tochihara, Y. and Ohnaka, T. (1999). Bathing before sleep in the young and in the elderly. European Journal of Applied Physiology and Occupational Physiology, 80(2), pp.71-75.

11. Jacobson, B., Boolani, A. and Smith, D. (2009). Changes in back pain, sleep quality, and perceived stress after introduction of new bedding systems. Journal of Chiropractic Medicine, 8(1), pp.1-8.

12. Effectiveness of a selected bedding system on quality of sleep, low back pain, shoulder pain, and spine stiffness

13. Libert, J., Bach, V., Johnson, L., Ehrhart, J., Wittersheim, G. and Keller, D. (1991). Relative and Combined Effects of Heat and Noise Exposure on Sleep in Humans. Sleep, 14(1), pp.24-31.

14. Higuchi, S., Motohashi, Y., Liu, Y. and Maeda, A. (2005). Effects of playing a computer game

using a bright display on presleep physiological variables, sleep latency, slow wave sleep and REM sleep. Journal of Sleep Research, 14(3), pp.267-273.

15. Rider, M., Floyd, J. and Kirkpatrick, J. (1985). The Effect of Music, Imagery, and Relaxation on Adrenal Corticosteroids and the Re-entrainment of Circadian Rhythms. Journal of Music Therapy, 22(1), pp.46-58.

16. Myllymaki T., Kyrolainen, H., Savolainen, K., Hokka, L., Jakonen, R., Juuti, T., Martinmaki, K., Kaartinen, J., Kinnunen, M. and Rusko, H. (2011). Effects of vigorous late-night exercise on sleep quality and cardiac autonomic activity. Journal of Sleep Research, 20(1pt2), pp.146-153.

17. Novak, C. and Levine, J. (2007). Central Neural and Endocrine Mechanisms of Non-Exercise Activity Thermogenesis and Their Potential Impact on Obesity. Journal of Neuroendocrinology, 19(12), pp.923-940.

18. Kaiser Permanente. "Keeping A Food Diary Doubles Diet Weight Loss, Study Suggests." ScienceDaily. ScienceDaily, 8 July 2008.

19. Pollock, R. (2016). The effect of green leafy and cruciferous vegetable intake on the incidence of cardiovascular disease: A meta-analysis. JRSM Cardiovascular Disease, 5, p.204800401666143.

20. White, C., Hitchcock, C., Vigna, Y. and Prior, J. (2011). Fluid Retention over the Menstrual Cycle: 1-Year Data from the Prospective Ovulation Cohort. Obstetrics and Gynecology International, 2011, pp.1-7.

21. McDonald, The Women's Book: Volume 1, A Guide to Nutrition, Fat Loss, and Muscle Gain, p 18).

22. Parr, E., Camera, D., Areta, J., Burke, L., Phillips, S., Hawley, J. and Coffey, V. (2014). Alcohol Ingestion Impairs Maximal Post-Exercise Rates of Myofibrillar Protein Synthesis following a Single Bout of Concurrent Training. PLoS ONE, 9(2), p.e88384.

23. Burke, L., Collier, G. and Hargreaves, M. (1996). Muscle Glycogen Storage Followed Prolonged Exercise: Effect Of Alcohol Intake 767. Medicine &amp Science in Sports &amp Exercise, 28(Supplement), p.129.

GLOSSARY

Aerobic pathway - The aerobic pathway is the process the body uses to create energy with the presence of oxygen (p.9, 30, 49)

Aerobic glycolysis - Aerobic glycolysis is the process the body uses to create energy from carbohydrates with the presence of oxygen (p.30, 32)

Amino acid - Amino acids are organic compounds that combine to form proteins (p.41-42, 63, 72, 74)

Anabolic hormonal profile - Anabolic hormones are insulin, testosterone are growth hormones, which are responsible for muscle mass and gains in strength (p.43)

Anaerobic glycolysis - Anaerobic glycolysis is the process our body uses to create energy from carbohydrates without the presence of oxygen (p.30, 32)

Anaerobic metabolism - Anaerobic metabolism is the way your body creates energy using carbohydrates, amino acids, and fats not in the presence of oxygen (p.9, 23, 31)

Antioxidants - Antioxidants are compounds that inhibit oxidation which is a process that may damage the cells of organisms (p. 51, 77)

ATP - Adenosine triphosphate provides energy to use in all bodily processes (p.8-10, 31, 33, 77)

Beta-oxidation - Beta oxidation is a metabolic process that breaks down fatty acids to produce energy (p.48)

Blood glucose - is the amount of glucose (sugar) in the blood (p.32, 48, 57-58, 60-61)

Body composition – body composition refers to the percentages of fat, bone, water and muscle in the body (p.22-25, 29-30, 36, 39-42, 44, 47, 82, 85-86, 88, 98-99, 102, 112, 115, 118-119, 127, 148, 156-158, 183)

BW – BW is a term used for body weight

Caloric intake - Caloric intake is as the amount of energy we consume via food and drink (p.29, 38, 43-44, 136, 192)

Carbohydrate availability – the availability of carbohydrates before, during and after exercise sessions to ensure there is enough energy to meet training demands (p.36, 43-44, 56, 58)

Carbohydrate mouth rinse - Carbohydrate (CHO) mouth rinse is swilling a carbohydrate solution around the mouth for 5 to 10s before spitting it out (p.37, 61, 68)

Carbohydrate periodisation - carbohydrate periodisation is the management of carbohydrates based around training (p.35, 38-39, 49)

CHO – another term used for carbohydrates (p.30)

Complex carbohydrates - complex carbohydrates are typically high in fibre (wholegrains, vegetables and fruit) and raise blood sugar levels slowly (p.38, 140-141)

Energy availability - Energy availability is the amount of dietary energy remaining after exercise training for all other metabolic processes (p.23, 53)

Energy balance - Energy balance refers to the amount of food and drink eaten compared to the number of kcals expended through activity (p.14-15)

Energy expenditure - Energy expenditure is the amount of energy or calories you burn or expend (p.16-17, 19, 21, 25, 41, 84, 111-120, 157)

Exercise capacity - Exercise capacity refers to how much physical exertion a person can withstand (p.8-9, 51, 59, 73, 76)

Fat oxidisation - Fat oxidation is use of fatty acids in the fat cell and in the blood for energy (p.31, 37)

g.kg.day– is a term used to express how much of a particular food, liquid or supplement we require. For example. If we require 2 grams of protein per kilogram per day we would say 2g.kg.day (p.41)

Glucose – glucose is sugar (p.32, 48, 57-58, 60-61)

Glycaemic index – glycaemic index refers to an index that is used to measure how quickly a carbohydrate food increases the level of glucose in the blood (p.45)

Glycogen - Glycogen is a form of carbohydrates stored for energy in humans (p.9, 31-38, 49, 57-62, 65-69, 104, 157, 183)

Glycogen depletion - Glycogen depletion is when we run out of glycogen stores (p.57, 60)

High GI carbohydrates - High GI carbohydrates are carbs that break down quickly (p.59, 65, 68-69)

Hypertrophy – Hypertrophy training refers to exercise used to increase muscle mass (p.32, 40)

Hyponatremia – Hyponatremia is low sodium levels in the blood (p.62)

IIFYM - If it fits your macros – This is a diet strategy which simply means eat what you like, providing you hit your macronutrient targets for the day (p.183)

Insulin – Insulin is a hormone that regulates the amount of glucose in the blood (p.46-48, 58, 84)

Kcal - A kcal or calorie is a unit of energy that is defined as the amount of heat energy required to raise 1 g of water by 1°C

Kcal balance – Kcal or energy balance is when there is a balance of kcals consumed through eating and drinking compared to kcals expended through activity (p.48, 184)

Kcal deficit - A kcal deficit is when the kcals consumed through food and drink are less than the kcals expended through exercise (p.14, 24, 83-89, 183)

Kcal maintenance – A kcal maintenance is the number of kcals required to maintain your current body weight (p.84-93, 115, 121, 152, 168-169)

Kcal surplus – A kcal surplus is the number of kcals required to increase your current body weight (p.15, 84-90, 168)

LCHF – Low carbohydrate high fat diet (p.31, 43-44)

Leucine - Leucine is an essential amino acid that is used in the production of proteins (p.41-45, 72)

Lipolysis - the breakdown of fats and other lipids by hydrolysis to release fatty acids (p.46-47)

Macronutrients - a type of food (e.g. fat, protein, carbohydrate) required in large amounts in the diet (p. 31-51)

Mediterranean diet - a diet of a type traditional in Mediterranean countries, characterized especially by a high consumption of vegetables and olive oil and moderate consumption of protein, and thought to lead to a number of health benefits (p.48)

MET – Metabolic equivalent. A MET is the ratio of the rate of energy expend-ed during an activity to the rate of energy expended at rest (p.20-25, 111, 115, 216)

Metabolic conditioning (Metcon) - Metabolic Conditioning is a method of training that involves a very high work rate, using exercises designed to burn more calories during your workout and maximise calories burned after your workout (p.8, 35, 92)

Metabolic dysfunction/Metabolic syndrome- are conditions that relate to cardiovascular disease, abdominal obesity, atherogenic dyslipidaemia, raised blood pressure, insulin resistance, glucose intolerance, proinflammatory and prothrombotic states (p.48)

Metabolism - Metabolism is the process of converting food to energy (p9-10, 23, 31)

MFP – MyFitnessPal - MyFitnessPal is a tracking app that can be used to track food intake (p.127-135)

MHR – Maximum heart rate - The maximum heart rate is how many beats your heart can beat per minute. To calculate your MHR subtract your age from 220 (p.112)

Micronutrients - Micronutrients are essential nutrients that are required in small quantities for the body to function correctly (p.52-56)

Mitochondria - Mitochondria is an organelle in the cell which produces energy (ATP) for the body to use (p.36-37)

Ml.kg.bw – millilitres per kilogram of bodyweight. This is a term used to express the amount of fluid an individual requires based on their weight (p.34, 59)

Muscle protein breakdown – Muscle protein breakdown is the process of muscle degradation (p.10, 40-41)

Muscle protein synthesis - Muscle protein synthesis is the process of building muscle tissue (p.41-42, 63, 72, 103)

NEAT – Non-exercise activity thermogenesis (NEAT) is the amount of energy expended during the day outside of structured exercise which include things like fidgeting and moving around (p.84, 103, 168)

Negative energy balance– A negative energy balance is similar to a kcal deficit, which indicates a deficiency in the number of kcals consumed compared to the number of kcals needed to maintain a set weight (p.14-15)

Overreaching - Overreaching is similar to overtraining but less severe and can be recovered from quickly (p.37)

Overtraining - Overtraining is when an individual is unable to recover properly from exercise

Oxidative stress - Oxidative stress is an imbalance of the number of free radicals and the body's ability to repair the resulting damage (p.51, 77)

PAL – The physical activity level (PAL) is a method to estimate an individual's energy expenditure (p.19, 25, 111, 114-121)

Paleo – The Paleo diet focuses on foods that were thought to be eaten by early humans, consisting mainly of meat, fish, vegetables, and fruit and excluding dairy and processed food (p.30, 48)

Periodisation - Periodised nutrition refers to the manipulation of nutrition to attain adaptations in the body that support performance (p.35, 38-39, 49)

Positive protein balance – A positive protein balance means that there is a larger intake of protein into the body than the loss of protein from the body (p.41)

Postprandial state – The postprandial dip is used to describe the decrease in blood sugar levels after eating (p.47)

The Postabsorptive State - The postabsorptive state is the period that's occurs once you have digested, absorbed and stored any food eaten (p.47)

Recommended daily allowance – RDA's – RDA's are the recommended amount of a nutrient or food group to maintain good health (p.50, 53, 190)

Upper respiratory tract infections – infections that include colds, the flu, tonsillitis, laryngitis, sinusitis, and the common cold (p.53)

RM – Rep max. 1RM stands for One Repetition Maximum. It is the maximum an individual can lift (p.10, 160)

Slow twitch muscle fibres - Slow twitch muscle fibres are suited to slower endurance-based activities (p.36)

TEA – Thermic effect of activity - Thermic effect of activity is the energy cost of all physical activity. This includes non-exercise activity (like fidgeting) along with structured exercise (p.16-17, 19)

TEE - Total Energy expenditure is the number of kcals expended by an individual during the day after accounting for activity and exercise (p.16-17)

Tempo – Tempo refers to the speed of the exercise being performed during resistance training (p.32, 161)

Training load - Training load is a way to measure the combination of volume and intensity of an individual's training (p.37)

Training low - Training low is training under low muscle glycogen conditions (p.36-37, 89, 97)

VO2 Max – VO2 Max is the maximum amount of oxygen your body can use during exercise and a way of measuring an individual's aerobic capacity (p.30-31, 60, 65, 68)

Volume - Volume refers to the amount of training being done (p.19-20, 23, 32-35, 41, 44-45, 49, 57, 64, 92, 112)

Zone diet - The Zone diet emphasises a low-carbohydrate approach to eating, however does not account for individual differences in training (p.30)